Practical
Veterinary
Urinalysis

Practical Veterinary Urinalysis

Carolyn A. Sink, MS, MT (ASCP)
Nicole M. Weinstein, DVM, DACVP
Illustrations by Ashley Marlowe

WILEY-BLACKWELL

A John Wiley & Sons, Inc., Publication

This edition first published 2012 © 2012 by John Wiley & Sons, Inc.

Wiley-Blackwell is an imprint of John Wiley & Sons, formed by the merger of Wiley's global Scientific, Technical and Medical business with Blackwell Publishing.

Registered office: John Wiley & Sons Ltd, The Atrium, Southern Gate, Chichester, West Sussex, PO19 8SQ, UK

Editorial offices: 2121 State Avenue, Ames, Iowa 50014-8300, USA
The Atrium, Southern Gate, Chichester, West Sussex, PO19 8SQ, UK
9600 Garsington Road, Oxford, OX4 2DQ, UK

For details of our global editorial offices, for customer services and for information about how to apply for permission to reuse the copyright material in this book please see our website at www.wiley.com/wiley-blackwell.

Library of Congress Cataloging-in-Publication Data

Sink, Carolyn A.
  Practical veterinary urinalysis / Carolyn Sink and Nicole Weinstein ; illustrations by Ashley Marlowe.
      p. ; cm.
  Includes bibliographical references and index.
  ISBN 978-0-470-95824-7 (pbk. : alk. paper)
  I. Weinstein, Nicole.   II. Title.
  [DNLM: 1. Urinalysis-veterinary-Laboratory Manuals. SF 773]
  LC classification not assigned
  636.089'66-dc23
                          2011035231

A catalogue record for this book is available from the British Library.

Wiley also publishes its books in a variety of electronic formats. Some content that appears in print may not be available in electronic books.

Set in 9 on 12.5 pt Interstate Light by Toppan Best-set Premedia Limited

Disclaimer

SKY10059101_110223

This book is dedicated to veterinary students, clinical laboratory professionals, clinical veterinarians, and all those who continue to develop and improve the veterinary clinical laboratory.

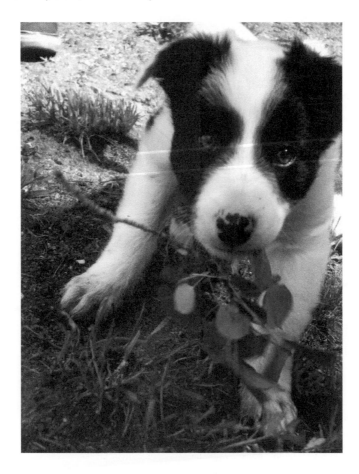

Contents

Preface

Laboratory evaluation of urine provides a significant amount of information to the veterinarian, as a variety of disease states may produce abnormal findings. Routine laboratory tests used to assess urine are quick and inexpensive, as well as reliable, when performed by a well-trained laboratory professional. *Practical Veterinary Urinalysis* is intended to provide laboratory diagnosticians—veterinarians, medical technologists, veterinary technicians, and veterinary students—with a comprehensive study of all aspects of routine urinalysis, including chemical analysis and microscopy. Those tasked with performing routine urinalysis will find both consolidated and comprehensive information needed to produce timely and accurate results.

Practical Veterinary Urinalysis is designed to provide the reader with a concise, systematic overview of renal physiology and urine production. Both functional and physiological aspects of the urinary system are reviewed with disease processes highlighted. When appropriate, discussions are reinforced by images, tables, and drawings. Specimen collection and handling are reviewed with emphasis on differences in laboratory findings between three frequently used methods.

An in-depth discussion of urine physical properties, chemical analysis, and sediment analysis is covered in separate chapters. Summarized charts are provided as testing guides when appropriate. Within the microscopic analysis section, *Practical Veterinary Urinalysis* contains images of the wet prep along with cytology (Wright's stain), and Gram stain if indicated.

Abnormal or suspicious results obtained by routine urinalysis may mandate additional or confirmatory tests. A chapter dedicated to advanced urine diagnostics presents newer test methodologies, and associated laboratory procedures are discussed.

Practical Veterinary Urinalysis also includes sections dedicated to laboratory setup, including physical and functional requirements along with instrument, reagent, and supply preferences. Quality assurance measures and quality goals are defined, assuring laboratorians that the results they produce are reliable.

Acknowledgments

We are grateful for the support and guidance of Drs. Rachel Cianciolo and Reema Patel, who provided invaluable insight and editorial commentary. We would also like to acknowledge veterinary students Rachel Baum and Alicyn Cross for their laboratory prowess in identifying interesting urine samples used in this book.

Carolyn Sink and Nicole Weinstein

Chapter 1

Functional Renal Physiology and Urine Production

Urinalysis can provide insight into hydration status, renal function or dysfunction, systemic disease, and toxic insults. Accurate interpretation of urinalysis results requires knowledge of renal physiology and urine formation.

Given the complexity of both, a brief overview is presented below; more detailed explanations can be found in a variety of references on which this chapter is based (Gregory 2003; Kaneko 2008; Schrier 2007; Stockham and Scott 2008; Watson 1998).

Descriptions of renal function and schematics of the kidney typically portray a single nephron, which is the functional unit of the kidney; each kidney contains hundreds of thousands of nephrons working in unison (Reece 1993). Each nephron requires:

(1) A blood supply
(2) A functional glomerulus, which filters a portion of the renal blood flow, to form an ultrafiltrate
(3) Renal tubules that function to reabsorb water, electrolytes, and other substances from the ultrafiltrate
(4) Collecting tubules and ducts, which further reabsorb or excrete water and solutes and thus determine final urine concentration.

Urine formation starts as an ultrafiltrate formed by glomerular filtration. The ultrafiltrate is then further altered by tubular reabsorption and secretion.

Glomerular filtration

The glomerulus is a collection of twisted capillaries that receive blood from the afferent arteriole of the renal blood supply and exit the kidney via the efferent arteriole (Figure 1.1). The high pressure within this system results in passage of fluids and small substances out of the capillaries into a space around the glomerulus, known as Bowman's capsule, which together form a renal corpuscle.

Practical Veterinary Urinalysis, First Edition. Carolyn Sink, Nicole Weinstein.
© 2012 John Wiley & Sons, Inc. Published 2012 by John Wiley & Sons, Inc.

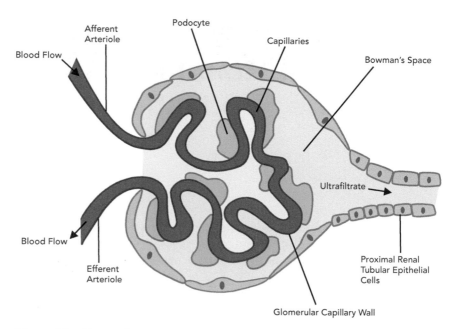

Figure 1.1 Glomerulus.

Glomerular filtration is driven by both blood volume and pressure and is considered a primarily passive process. Ultrafiltrate is the product of glomerular filtration of blood following its passage through a glomerular filtration barrier, the glomerular capillary wall (GCW). The GCW prevents entry of red and white blood cells, platelets, and larger proteins into the ultrafiltrate. The exact composition and function of the GCW is the subject of intense research and debate currently in the human literature. Additional information is presented about glomerular filtration and the GCW in Chapter 6, "Proteinuria."

Concentrations of urea, creatinine, amino acids, glucose, bicarbonate, and electrolytes are similar between the ultrafiltrate and plasma. Specific gravity (SG) which ranges from 1.008 to 1.012 and osmolality (300 mOsm/kg with a range of 280-310 mOsm/kg) will also be similar between the two (Watson 1998). Note the SG range of 1.008-1.012 is identical to the range described for isosthenuria. For additional information regarding interpretation of urine specific gravity (USG), see Chapter 3. Knowledge of this range is relevant for the diagnosis of renal failure as well as the interpretation of urine with an SG of less than 1.008. Chapter 3, "Routine Urinalysis: Physical Properties," discusses USG in greater detail.

Renal blood flow ultimately determines the glomerular filtration rate (GFR) or rate of blood flow within the glomerulus. GFR can be affected by numerous factors such as a patient's blood volume, cardiac output, and total number of functional glomeruli (Stockham and Scott 2008). GFR and direct and indirect measures of GFR can therefore be influenced by renal disease as well

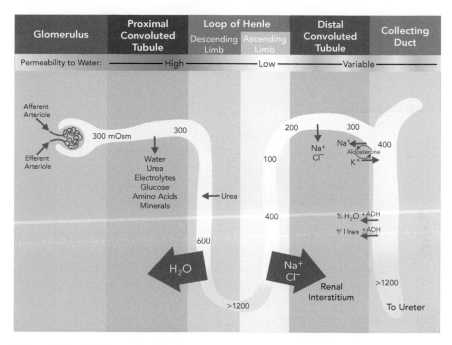

Figure 1.2 Solute and water handling in the renal tubule.
Source: Gregory (2003); Kaneko (2008); Stockham and Scott (2008).

as nonrenal factors such as dehydration, severe blood loss, hypotension, diuretic use, fluid therapy, and hypoalbuminemia to name a few.

Ultrafiltrate exiting Bowman's capsule enters into the proximal convoluted tubule (PCT).

Tubular reabsorption and secretion

Tubular reabsorption and secretion employ both passive and active mechanisms to ultimately form urine, conserve water and necessary solutes, and excrete waste products. The renal tubules are divided into the PCT, ascending and descending loops of Henle, distal convoluted tubule, and the collecting duct. Each segment serves to reabsorb and/or secrete water and various solutes (Figure 1.2). Reabsorption serves to prevent water and solutes from being excreted into the tubular fluid while secretion results in loss of either into the tubular fluid. Water and solutes remaining in the tubular fluid are excreted as urine.

Proximal convoluted tubule

The majority of water and solutes are reabsorbed in the PCT. Sodium is actively reabsorbed in the PCT via several mechanisms and water follows passively. In addition to sodium reabsorption, conservation of amino acids, glucose, phosphate, chloride, potassium, and bicarbonate occurs in the PCT. Fluid in the PCT displays only mild increases in SG and osmolality relative to the ultrafiltrate. Ultimately, water conservation reduces the volume of tubular fluid by 70% (Kaneko 2008; Stockham and Scott 2008; Watson 1998).

Loop of Henle

The loop of Henle includes a descending loop and ascending loop that serve to reabsorb more water and electrolytes through both passive and active mechanisms. The renal medullary interstitium, which is the tissue and fluid surrounding the tubules, and peritubular capillaries are integral parts of the conservation of water and electrolytes.

The descending loop of Henle is permeable to water but is impermeable to electrolytes. As the loop descends into the renal medulla, which is maintained at a higher osmolality due to higher concentrations of both sodium and urea, the water will exit the loop in an attempt to equilibrate with the surrounding interstitium, thus serving to conserve water. As water exits the tubular fluid, the osmolality and SG greatly increase as the tubular fluid prepares to enter the ascending loop.

The ascending loop of Henle is opposite to the descending loop and is permeable to urea and electrolytes (mostly sodium, chloride, and potassium) but impermeable to water. Tubular fluid ascends the loop of Henle and becomes increasingly more dilute as sodium and chloride are first passively and then actively reabsorbed into the medullary interstitium. Medullary interstitial hypertonicity results from the increase in sodium concentration.

Blood vessels, specifically peritubular capillaries that parallel the loop of Henle, are termed the "vasa recta." Blood in the vasa recta flows in the opposite direction to the fluid in the loop of Henle. The loop of Henle, together with the vasa recta and interstitium, comprise a countercurrent system. The process of countercurrent multiplication is essential in maintaining a concentration gradient within the medullary interstitium as both the descending loop of Henle and collecting ducts require a hypertonic medullary interstitium for water reabsorption. Therefore, the hypertonicity of the medullary interstitium is a product of the descending loop of Henle as described above. A basic understanding of this gradient aids in interpreting extrarenal influences on urine concentration and will be discussed below (Gregory 2003; Kaneko 2008; Schrier 2007; Stockham and Scott 2008; Watson 1998).

Distal (convoluted) tubule

The epithelial cells of the distal tubule demonstrate minimal permeability to water. Sodium and chloride, however, can be reabsorbed from the tubular fluid in this segment primarily under the influence of aldosterone, antidiuretic hormone (ADH), and other substances.

Collecting tubules

Although the majority of water and solute reabsorption occurs in the PCT and loop of Henle, the collecting tubules determine the final urine volume and USG. The collecting tubule is impermeable to water except in the presence of ADH, which results in reabsorption of water. ADH levels ultimately determine whether urine will be dilute or concentrated. High concentrations of urea, sodium, or chloride in the medullary interstitium facilitate ADH reabsorption of water, again reinforcing the necessity of a hypertonic renal medullary interstitium. In the absence of ADH, dilute urine is produced.

Renal function and measures of renal function

In the normal state, the goal of the kidneys is to conserve water, glucose, amino acids, sodium, chloride, bicarbonate, calcium, magnesium, and most proteins, and to excrete urea, creatinine, phosphate, potassium, hydrogen ions, ammonium, ketones, bilirubin, hemoglobin, and myoglobin (Stockham and Scott 2008). Additional roles of the kidneys include, but are not limited to, erythropoietin synthesis to stimulate red blood cell development, acid-base regulation, renin secretion, calcium and phosphorous homeostasis, and blood pressure regulation. Urea nitrogen (UN) and creatinine are both waste products of metabolism and are filtered and excreted by the kidneys into the urine.

Urea production and excretion

The liver converts ammonia, which is a product of intestinal protein catabolism, into urea. Urea, following release by the liver into the blood, is freely filtered by the glomerulus and enters the ultrafiltrate. Urea follows water into and out of the renal tubules. The amount of urea excreted in the urine varies from 40% to 70% of the ultrafiltrate and is mostly determined by flow rate within the tubules (Schrier 2007). At higher urine flow rates (i.e. increased water or fluid intake), less urea is reabsorbed and so more is excreted in the urine. Decreased urine flow rate (i.e. dehydration) results in a greater amount of urea reabsorption and so less is excreted into the urine.

Creatinine excretion

Creatinine is produced at a constant rate from normal muscle metabolism where creatine in muscle is converted to creatinine (Gregory 2003; Kaneko 2008; Stockham and Scott 2008). Creatine concentrations are influenced by an animal's muscle mass and underlying disease states. Similar to urea, creatinine is freely filtered by the glomerulus, meaning it passes through the glomerular filtration barrier and enters into the tubular fluid. In contrast to urea, creatinine is not reabsorbed by the renal tubules. A small amount of creatinine, however, is excreted by the proximal tubule in male dogs.

Laboratory assessment of renal function

Urea and creatinine concentrations are the most commonly utilized tests to evaluate renal function. Urea concentration, typically measured in serum or plasma, is reported as UN or blood urea nitrogen (BUN). The amount of urea in whole blood, serum, or plasma is identical because urea rapidly equilibrates between compartments. Because of the variability in the amount of urea presented to the kidney and the potential for tubular reabsorption of urea, both nonrenal and renal factors influence BUN. Creatinine is a more accurate measure of GFR given its constant rate of formation and lack of tubular reabsorption (Kaneko 2008; Stockham and Scott 2008).

Azotemia

An increase in BUN and creatinine is termed azotemia. Azotemia can be prerenal, renal, or postrenal in origin although causes may be multifactorial. Prerenal azotemia results from decreased renal blood flow. Examples of prerenal azotemia include hypovolemia due to dehydration or hemorrhage, shock, decreased cardiac output, hypotension, and so on. Concentrated urine (USG > 1.030 in dogs and >1.035 in cats) is an expected finding with prerenal azotemia. Renal azotemia can be due to acute or chronic renal failure as a result of greater than 75% loss of functioning glomeruli. Renal azotemia results in inadequately concentrated urine (USG < 1.030 in dogs and <1.035 in cats); isosthenuria (USG 1.008–1.012) in the face of azotemia is indicative of renal disease. Postrenal azotemia is caused by obstructed urine flow from urethral or ureteral obstruction (i.e. urinary calculi), bladder rupture, neoplasia, neurologic disease, or congenital abnormalities. The USG can vary with postrenal azotemia. BUN and creatinine concentrations tend to parallel one another in renal and postrenal causes of azotemia. Increases in BUN without a concomitant increase in creatinine or a disproportionally higher increase in BUN relative to the increase in creatinine can be seen in certain prerenal conditions, that is, increased protein catabolism and dehydration. As described earlier, diminished renal tubular flow rate and the presence of ADH both increase urea reabsorption by the renal tubules and can elevate BUN. Increased protein catabolism, especially in animals fed a high-protein diet or with small intestinal bleeding, can result in elevated BUN (Table 1.1).

Decreased BUN can hinder renal concentrating ability. Urea contributes approximately half of the hypertonicity of the renal medullary interstitial fluid, which facilitates water reabsorption from the tubular fluid. Decreased BUN can result from hepatic failure or shunting of hepatic blood flow away from the liver (i.e. portosystemic shunt) so that ammonia cannot be converted into urea. Increased renal excretion of urea can also decrease BUN such as with excess glucose in the renal tubular fluid (i.e. diabetes mellitus) or very high renal tubular flow rates. Low BUN can then result in a lower than expected USG even in a dehydrated patient. BUN value should be considered

Table 1.1 Pre-renal causes of an increased BUN

Increased protein catabolism
Fever
Starvation
Corticosteriods
High protein diet
Prolonged exercise
Small intestinal hemorrhage

Decreased excretion due to decreased renal blood flow*
Shock
Hypotension
Decreased cardiac output (e.g., heart failure)
Hypovolemia (dehydration, hemorrhage, hypoadrenocorticism)

* May also cause increase in serum creatinine concentration.
Source: Gregory (2003); Stockham and Scott (2008)

when interpreting USG. Similarly, low plasma concentrations of sodium and chloride, termed hyponatremia and hypochloremia, respectively, can also diminish renal concentrating function due to a less hypertonic renal medullary interstitium.

Although routine, BUN and creatinine are relatively insensitive measures of renal function. Renal azotemia does not develop until after 75% or greater functional nephrons are lost or damaged. In renal failure, the diseased kidneys cannot adequately excrete urea or creatinine. Postrenal causes of azotemia also result in an inability to excrete urea and creatinine from the body. Determination of prerenal, renal, and postrenal causes of azotemia utilize USG as well as historical, physical exam, and other clinicopathological data.

Osmolality

Osmolality is the concentration of solutes in a solution (Kaneko 2008; Stockham and Scott 2008; Watson 1998). The largest contributors to plasma osmolality are sodium, urea, and glucose (Stockham and Scott 2008). Plasma osmolality is sensed by receptors in the hypothalamus. Plasma osmolality and osmolality within the renal tubular fluid and medullary interstitium, as described above, impact urine formation. Increased plasma osmolality results in ADH release, which stimulates the collecting tubules and ducts to reabsorb water. The opposite is true of decreased osmolality. With low plasma osmolality, ADH is not secreted and more water is excreted into the urine.

In conclusion, renal physiology is a complex and elaborate process. This chapter provides only a brief summary of basic renal function so as to facilitate understanding of the physiologic processes that impact and determine urine formation and to maximize interpretation of urinalysis.

Chapter 1

References

Gregory CR. 2003. Urinary system. In *Duncan & Prasse's Veterinary Laboratory Medicine Clinical Pathology*, 4th ed. Latimer KS, Mahaffe EA, Prasse KW, eds., pp. 231-59. Ames, IA: Iowa State Press.

Kaneko JJ. 2008. Kidney function and damage. In *Clinical Biochemistry of Domestic Animals*, 6th ed. Kaneko JJ, Harvey JW, Bruss ML, eds., pp. 485-528. Burlington, VT: Elsevier Inc.

Reece WO. 1993. The kidneys. In *Dukes' Physiology of Domestic Animals*, 11th ed. Swenson MJ, Reece WO, eds., pp. 573-603. Ithaca, NY: Cornell University Press.

Schrier RW. 2007. Laboratory evaluation of kidney function. In *Diseases of the Kidney and Urinary Tract*, vol. 1, 8th ed. Schrier RW, ed., pp. 299-366. Philadelphia: Lippincott Williams & Wilkins.

Stockham SL, Scott MA. 2008. Urinary system. In *Fundamentals of Veterinary Clinical Pathology*, 2nd ed. Stockham SL, Scott MA, eds., pp. 415-94. Ames, IA: Blackwell Publishing.

Watson ADJ. 1998. Urine specific gravity in practice. *Australian Veterinary Journal* **76**(6): 392-8.

Chapter 2
Specimen Procurement

Urinalysis test results are influenced by many preanalytical variables, the majority of which can be controlled during urine specimen collection. This chapter reviews common methods of urine collection, appropriate use of urine specimen containers and urine preservation techniques, and the potential impact of each on urinalysis results. Minimizing these preanalytical variables will allow for the most consistent and reliable urinalysis results.

Laboratory definitions for collection methods

An overview of collection methods may be found in Table 2.1.

Voided or "free catch"

Natural micturition is the least invasive method of collecting urine (Wamsley and Alleman 2007). Ideally, urine is collected midstream as first-stream urine is more likely to contain bacteria, cells, and other debris from the vulva, urethra, or prepuce. To further minimize contamination, the patient's urogenital area can be cleansed prior to specimen collection and a sterile container can be used to catch the urine. Free-catch samples are most at risk for contamination by the genital tract, skin, or hair, which can result in a false-positive urine bacterial culture (Osborne and Stevens 1999). If the only urine sample available for culture is a free-catch sample, quantitative analysis should be performed (Reine and Langston 2005).

For an inexperienced person, timing the collection of a voided urine sample from a dog can be tricky as the collection attempt may cause the animal to cease urinating. Some recommend a long-handled ladle or shallow pie tin to collect urine from a female dog or a large cup to collect urine from a male dog (Mathes 2002). Collecting a free catch, midstream urine sample from a cat is also challenging. Urine can be obtained from a clean litter box or one

Practical Veterinary Urinalysis, First Edition. Carolyn Sink, Nicole Weinstein.
© 2012 John Wiley & Sons, Inc. Published 2012 by John Wiley & Sons, Inc.

Table 2.1 Advantages and disadvantages of urine collection methods

Method of Collection	Pro	Con
Free-catch	No risk to the patient Easy to perform Can be used to localize lesion	Unsuitable for bacterial culture Contaminants common Subject to patient's need to urinate
Manual expression	None	Risk of bladder injury Possible reflux of urine into kidneys, prostate Difficult to impossible in awake patients
Catheterization	Lower risk of contamination Relatively safe for the patient	Technical skill required Often requires sedation Challenging in a patient with obstruction
Cystocentesis	Best sample for bacterial culture Can be performed in awake patient Relatively safe	Technical skill required Blood contamination in sample Increased risk to patient for hemorrhage, bladder rupture Avoid in patient with coagulopathy

lined with a clean trash bag; no absorbent litter is used. An option for cats that refuse to use a litter-free litter box is to add a nonabsorbable material such as Nosorb® beads (Catco, Inc., Cape Coral, FL) or packing peanuts (Styrofoam™, Midland, MI, or plastic). Urine collected by these methods would be unsuitable for bacterial cultures given the many potential sources for contamination although physical and chemical properties should remain valid. The urine should be collected from the litter box promptly so as to minimize crystal formation and potential increases in urine specific gravity (USG) (Albasan et al. 2003; Steinberg et al. 2009).

Table collection

Recovering urine from the floor or exam table is occasionally a necessity as patients, due to fear or excitement, may urinate unexpectedly. This is essentially a free-catch sample with additional sources of contamination from the site where the urine is collected. Bacteria, hyphal structures, and foreign material, if identified, should be considered as such and another sample collected, especially if bacterial culture is needed. Cleaning agents used to clean various surfaces in the hospital or clinic can result in false-positive dipstick reactions for protein, glucose, blood, or leukocyte esterase (Strasinger and DiLorenzo 2008).

Manual expression of the bladder

This method of urine collection is subject to many of the same considerations as free-catch urine samples. In an awake animal, however, manual expression is not advised (Reine and Langston 2005) as the pressure necessary to induce micturition can result in reflux of urine (vesicoureteral reflux), potentially containing bacteria from the genital tract, into the ureters, renal pelves, kidneys, and, in male dogs, the prostate. Urinary bladder expression is contra-indicated in patients with a urinary outflow obstruction or recent cystotomy.

Urinary catheterization

Catheterization of the urinary bladder is another method of urine collection and can be used in both cats and dogs; it obviously requires a greater degree of technical skill than a urine sample obtained by free catch. Sterile technique should be followed both for the patient's urinary tract health and integrity of bacterial culture. Male dogs can often be catheterized awake; the majority of female dogs and both male and female cats must be sedated or anesthetized prior to urinary catheterization. For a detailed description and instructions for urinary catheterization and selection of urinary catheters, the reader is directed to other resources (Reine and Langston 2005). Briefly, the external genitalia should be cleansed prior to catheterization and only sterile lubricant and sterilized catheter, instruments, and syringe used (Barsanti 1984; Reine and Langston 2005). In the male, the prepuce should be retracted and the tip of the penis cleaned with dilute chlorhexiderm solution prior to insertion of a sterile, lubricated, catheter into the urethra (Reine and Langston 2005). Once the catheter is inserted into the urethra, it is advanced into the bladder; a sterile syringe is attached to the distal end of the catheter and is used to withdraw urine. Catheters should be selected based on the species as well as the patient size and gender. When collected using a sterile technique, bacterial contamination should be minimal to absent. The distal urethra, however, contains some normal bacterial flora that can contaminate the collected urine and confound bacterial culture results (Barsanti 1984). Increased numbers of squamous epithelial cells may also be seen in urine collected by catheterization. Discarding the first portion of urine specimen collected may minimize numbers of epithelial cells and/or bacteria.

For patients with indwelling urinary catheters, urine is collected in the same manner as described above, through a sterile syringe attached to the distal end of the catheter. The risk of bacterial infection in these patients, however, increases with duration of catheterization warranting bacterial culture in addition to urinalysis (Bubenik et al. 2007).

Cystocentesis

Cystocentesis is ideal for collecting urine samples for bacterial culture and is considered a valuable diagnostic tool (Kruger et al. 1996). It can usually be performed on an awake patient. The patient is placed in dorsal recumbency, and the skin of the ventral abdomen should be cleaned prior to each cysto-centesis attempt. In patients with abundant hair or fur, a small area should be clipped. The bladder can be located either manually or with ultrasound, if available; a bladder containing minimal urine may be difficult to detect. The bladder can be palpated and immobilized by the palpating hand or immobi-lized against the pelvis while the other hand is used to obtain the sample (Barsanti 1984; Reine and Langston 2005). For cystocentesis in cats, immo-bilization of the bladder by "gently grasping the neck of the bladder between the thumb and forefinger or compressing the bladder against the pelvic brim" is recommended (Barsanti 1984; Kruger et al. 1996; Reine and Langston 2005).

Following immobilization, the needle, attached to a syringe, is inserted, at an oblique angle, approximately 45°, through the wall of the ventral abdomen and is advanced caudally toward the pelvic inlet (Barsanti 1984; Kruger et al. 1996; Reine and Langston 2005). By angling the needle caudally, the needle will remain in the bladder lumen even as the bladder empties (Kruger et al. 1996; Reine and Langston 2005). Excessive digital pressure on the bladder should be avoided while the needle is inserted into the lumen so as to prevent leakage of urine around the needle site (Kruger et al. 1996). Urine can be aspirated slowly via the attached syringe. Cystocentesis is best in a patient with a somewhat distended bladder but not overly distended or obstructed urinary bladder. Release pressure on the bladder prior to removal of the needle from the bladder.

Depending on patient size, a 21-gauge (or smaller) 1 to 1.5-inch needle is preferred; a 6–12 mL syringe is typically used (Kruger et al. 1996; Reine and Langston 2005). Very large or obese dogs may necessitate the use of a longer needle, that is, 1.5–2 inches (Reine and Langston 2005).

Although cystocentesis is generally considered safe, it is not entirely without risk. Mild to moderate hematuria is the most common side effect and may reflect the needle contacting the opposite wall of the bladder (Reine and Langston 2005). Uncommon but potential negative sequelae to cystocentesis include rupture of an overly distended bladder, peritonitis secondary to leakage of septic urine, laceration of the bladder wall, laceration of a major vessel, and inadvertent puncture of the large intestine (Buckley et al. 2009; Reine and Langston 2005). The presence of numerous mixed bacteria in the urine sample would suggest sampling from the intestine.

Urine specimen containers

Urine collection containers

Collection cups and devices are available in a variety of shapes and sizes and are selected based on the collection method utilized and anticipated sample size. While leak-resistant sample cups with snap or screw lid are

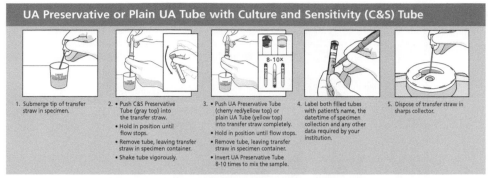

Figure 2.1 BD Vacutainer® collection product utilizing transfer straw for urine samples. (Provided by BD Diagnostics, with permission)

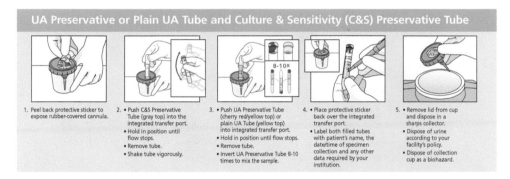

Figure 2.2 BD Vacutainer® collection product utilizing transfer cup for urine samples. (Provided by BD Diagnostics, with permission)

conventionally used for urine collection and transport, specialized urine collection-transport containers are commercially available that provide a unique approach to sample acquisition (Figures 2.1–2.4).

Urine containers for laboratory analysis

Depending on the urine collection method employed, urine samples are often transferred from the collection container to a secondary container to accommodate laboratory analysis. When selecting a secondary container, consideration should be given to the type of laboratory test(s) that will be performed on the urine sample. For example, the secondary container must fit into the centrifuge head that is used to acquire sediment for microscopic analysis. If microbial assessment is required in addition to urinalysis testing, all containers must be sterile. Sterile containers are also recommended if the urine specimen will not be analyzed within 1 hour of collection.

Any container employed must be break resistant, leakproof, and clean. Containers cannot be washed and reused as detergents interfere with chemical analysis and microscopic evaluation; artifacts can be acquired through improper washing, chemical residue, or other contaminants. Flat bottom containers prevent inadvertent overturning (Strasinger and DiLorenzo 2008).

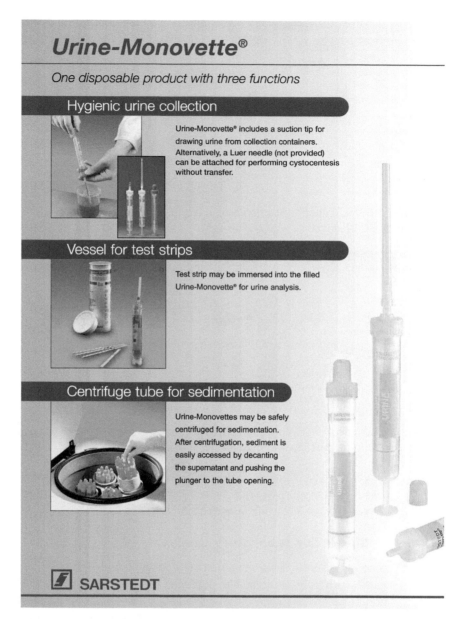

Figure 2.3 Sarstedt urine collection and testing product. (Provided by Sarstedt, with permission)

The container should not leach interfering substances or particles into the urine sample, and the exterior of the container must possess enough surface area for labeling. To expedite evaluation of physical characteristics, a clear container is mandatory. Tubes must withstand centrifugation, and if an automated system is used, compatibility with the loading rack or carrier is necessary.

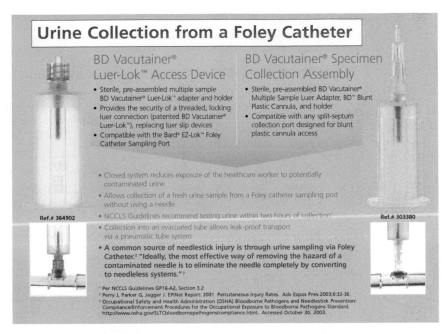

Figure 2.4 Catheter collection devices. (Provided by BD Diagnostics, with permission)

Specimen handling and preservation

Urine samples should be delivered to the laboratory and analyzed as soon as possible; recent literature suggests analysis of urine within 1 hour of collection (Albasan et al. 2003). Considerations include deterioration of cellular components and alterations in biochemical tests. The presence of bacteria in urine, either secondary to contamination or a result of a urinary tract infection, can result in a falsely negative urine glucose, due to bacterial overgrowth and metabolism of glucose, and falsely elevated urine pH, due to bacteria that split urea and convert it to ammonia. pH can also alter other cellular components in urine; alkaline urine can cause degradation of casts as well as lysis of erythrocytes, the latter resulting in a potential false interpretation of pigmenturia or hemoglobinemia rather than hematuria (Ben-Ezra et al. 2007; Osborne and Stevens 1999; Strasinger and DiLorenzo 2008).

There is no substitute for fresh urine. If a delay in testing is imminent, the urine specimen should be refrigerated. Refrigeration is the most commonly used method of urine preservation. Although refrigeration can better preserve cellular components and delay bacterial proliferation, it can result in some unintended effects. Refrigeration can result in an increased USG because cold urine is denser than room temperature urine. The cold temperature of the urine may inhibit enzyme reactions on the urine dipstick. Lastly, refrigeration can cause precipitation of amorphous crystals. Warming the specimen to room temperature prior to testing can ameliorate enzyme

Table 2.2 Common urine preservatives

Preservation Method	Pros	Cons
Refrigeration	Preserves chemical and formed elements Inhibits bacterial growth	Increases specific gravity Precipitates amorphous urates/phosphates
Formalin	Preserves sediment	Interferes with dipstick tests: glucose, blood, leukocyte esterase
Sodium fluoride	Inhibits glycolysis	Interferes with dipstick tests: glucose, blood, leukocyte esterase

reactions and dissolve crystal artifact (Ben-Ezra et al. 2007; Osborne and Stevens 1999; Strasinger and DiLorenzo 2008).

Although not recommended for routine urinalysis, sample integrity can be maintained by the addition of chemical preservatives; this may be necessary for samples needing extended transport when refrigeration is not an option. The appropriate preservative should not alter urine constituents or interfere with analytical test methodologies (Table 2.2).

Types of urine specimens

Random

The random specimen is the most common type of urine sample evaluated both in the veterinary clinic and clinical laboratory. As urine is frequently collected on an as-needed basis or is collected when readily available, several variables must be taken into consideration. Recent dietary or water intake, physical activity, total time urine has resided in the bladder, and recent therapeutic interventions can result in altered urine constituents leading to test results that may not accurately reflect the patient's current health status. For example, water intake can decrease specific gravity of the urine, diluting chemical constituents and lysing cellular elements. More controlled conditions for urine collection is often preferred for definitive diagnosis.

First morning or 8 hour

A urine sample collected immediately upon awakening is known as the first morning or 8-hour sample. First morning specimens are the most concentrated urine sample, allowing for evaluation of renal concentrating ability as well as detection of chemicals or formed elements that may not be easily measured in a more dilute, random urine sample. It is presumed that the animal has neither voided nor ingested food or water during the previous 8 hours while it has been asleep.

Fasting or second morning

Urine collected after a period of food deprivation is known as fasting or second morning sample. It should not contain metabolites from dietary ingestion.

Timed or 24-hour specimen

A 24-hour excretion study is used to determine urinary excretion of an analyte, such as electrolytes or protein, and is considered the most definitive method of measurement (Stockham and Scott 2008). Urine is collected for a 24-hour period; timing starts after the bladder is completely emptied (Stockham and Scott 2008). Collection of a 24-hour urine sample is, however, impractical in veterinary medicine for several reasons. It necessitates use of a metabolism cage to guarantee collection of all urine produced by an animal (Adams et al. 1992). Interpretation of laboratory results is dependent on reference ranges that are not always available for all species; reference ranges may be biased depending on the assay used or the type of diet the patient eats (Stockham and Scott 2008). In lieu of 24-hour urine collection, either urine to plasma ratio or analyte to creatinine ratio is used (Stockham and Scott 2008).

References

Adams LG, Polzin DJ, Osborne CA, O'Brien TD. 1992. Correlation of urine protein/creatinine ratio and twenty-four-hour urinary protein excretion in normal cats and cats with surgically induced chronic renal failure. *Journal of Veterinary Internal Medicine* **6**(1): 36-40.

Albasan H, Lulich JP, Osborne CA, Lekcharoensuk C, Ulrich LK, Carpenter KA. 2003. Effects of storage time and temperature on pH, specific gravity, and crystal formation in urine samples from dogs and cats. *Journal of the American Veterinary Medical Association* **222**(2): 176-9.

Barsanti JA. 1984. Diagnostic procedures in urology. *Veterinary Clinics of North America. Small Animal Practice* **14**(1): 3-14.

Ben-Ezra J, Zhao S, McPherson R. 2007. Basic examination of urine. In *Henry's Clinical Diagnosis and Management by Laboratory Methods*, 21st ed. McPherson RA, Pincus MR, eds., pp. 393-409. Philadelphia: Saunders Elsevier.

Bubenik LJ, Hosgood GL, Waldron DR, Snow LA. 2007. Frequency of urinary tract infection in catheterized dogs and comparison of bacterial culture and susceptibility testing results for catheterized and noncatheterized dogs with urinary tract infections. *Journal of the American Veterinary Medical Association* **231**(6): 893-9.

Buckley GJ, Aktay SA, Rozanski EA. 2009. Massive transfusion and surgical management of iatrogenic aortic laceration associated with cystocentesis in a dog. *Journal of the American Veterinary Medical Association* **235**(3): 288-91.

Kruger JM, Osborne CA, Ulrich LK. 1996. Cystocentesis. Diagnostic and therapeutic considerations. *Veterinary Clinics of North America. Small Animal Practice* **26**(2): 353-61.

Mathes MA. 2002. Home monitoring of the diabetic pet. *Clinical Techniques in Small Animal Practice* **17**(2): 86-95.

Osborne CA, Stevens JB. 1999. *Urinalysis: A Clinical Guide to Compassionate Patient Care.* Shawnee Mission, KS: Bayer Corporation.

Reine NJ, Langston CE. 2005. Urinalysis interpretation: how to squeeze out the maximum information from a small sample. *Clinical Techniques in Small Animal Practice* **20**(1): 2-10.

Steinberg E, Drobatz K, Aronson L. 2009. The effect of substrate composition and storage time on urine specific gravity in dogs. *Journal of Small Animal Practice* **50**(10)1:536-9.

Stockham SL, Scott MA. 2008. Urinary system. In *Fundamentals of Veterinary Clinical Pathology*, 2nd ed. Stockham SL, Scott MA, eds., pp. 415-94. Ames, IA: Blackwell Publishing.

Strasinger SK, DiLorenzo MS. 2008. Introduction to urinalysis. In *Urinalysis and Body Fluids*, 5th ed. Strasinger SK, DiLorenzo MS, eds., pp. 29-40. Philadelphia: FA Davis Company.

Wamsley H, Alleman R. 2007. Complete urinalysis. In *BSAVA Manual of Canine and Feline Nephrology and Urology*, 2nd ed. Elliot J, Grauer GF, eds., pp. 87-104. Gloucester: British Small Animal Veterinary Association.

Chapter 2

Chapter 3

Routine Urinalysis: Physical Properties

A basic but essential component of routine urinalysis is assessment of the physical properties of urine: color, clarity, specific gravity, and odor. This chapter reviews methods of specific gravity measurement as well as interpretation of urine specific gravity (USG), urine color, and clarity.

Solute concentration

Specific gravity

Specific gravity is one of two methods of measurement of urine solute concentration; the other measure is urine osmolality. Urine solutes are composed of numerous electrolytes as well as products of metabolism (urea and creatinine), which are excreted by the kidneys (Stockham and Scott 2008). Urine is composed of approximately 5% solutes and 95% water; solute concentration is affected by the hydration status of the patient (Figure 3.1). For example, when the kidneys must conserve water in a dehydrated patient, the urine solute concentration would be expected to increase as the amount of free water in the urine decreases. Solute number, size, and weight all influence the specific gravity of a urine sample. Larger particles such as urea, glucose, or proteins can increase USG readings more so than sodium or chloride. (See Chapter 1 for a detailed discussion of urine formation and tubular function.)

Measurement of specific gravity

To understand measurement of specific gravity, it may be easier to consider it a relative density, as it is a comparison of the weight of a solution to the weight of an equal volume of water. (Free 1987; Stockham and Scott 2008; Strasinger and DiLorenzo 2008)

Practical Veterinary Urinalysis, First Edition. Carolyn Sink, Nicole Weinstein.
© 2012 John Wiley & Sons, Inc. Published 2012 by John Wiley & Sons, Inc.

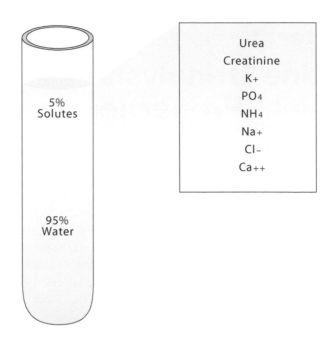

| Urea |
| Creatinine |
| K+ |
| PO₄ |
| NH₄ |
| Na+ |
| Cl– |
| Ca++ |

Figure 3.1 Normal urine composition.

Direct measurement

Direct measurement of specific gravity is possible but not practical for clinical purposes. Laboratory methods include urinometry and falling drop method.

Indirect measurement

Refractometry

Refractometry is an indirect method of USG determination and is based on the refractive index of urine. Refractometry has replaced direct methods of USG determination as refractometry is simple to perform, is relatively inexpensive, and provides a satisfactory estimate of USG when compared to direct methods such as urinometry.

The refractive index of a solution is the degree to which light waves entering the solution are bent or refracted by the solutes or substances present (Stockham and Scott 2008; Strasinger and DiLorenzo 2008; Watson 1998). Increasing amounts of solute in a solution cause the light to slow and refract proportionally to the amount of solutes present; this increases the refractive index. Thus, specific gravity of urine will increase with increasing solute concentration as it is the ratio of the refractive index of urine compared to water (Gregory 2003; Stockham and Scott 2008; Watson 1998). Glucosuria and proteinuria can both impact USG, resulting in overestimation of the USG. Protein concentration of 1g/dL (3+ for Chemstrip® 10 MD, Indianapolis, IN;

Idexx UA™ dry reagent strips, Westbrook, ME; 4+ for Multistix®, Tarrytown, NY) increases USG approximately 0.003–0.005 (Stockham and Scott 2008). Glucose concentration of 1000 mg/dL increases USG approximately 0.004–0.005 (Stockham and Scott 2008). Suspended particles such as casts, crystals, or cells do not refract light and so do not directly affect the refractive index or USG (Goldberg 1997). Light transmission, however, can be affected by particle-induced turbidity, which can hinder visualization of the demarcation line in the refractometer, potentially resulting in an erroneous result (Stockham and Scott 2008).

Along with solute concentration and composition, temperature can influence the refractive index (Stockham and Scott 2008) and thus the USG. Handheld refractometers are commonly used in veterinary practices, and automatic temperature compensation (ATC), manual temperature compensation, or no temperature compensation models are available (Ben-Ezra et al. 2007; George 2001; Strasinger and DiLorenzo 2008). Temperature compensation increases the expense of the unit but generally gives accurate readings between 60 and 100°F (16–38°C). For readings obtained with ATC refractometers, no mathematical temperature correction is necessary since the light beam passes through a temperature compensating liquid prior to being directed to the specific gravity scale, provided the reading is obtained within manufacturer-specified ambient temperature range. Refractometers that are not temperature compensated tend to underestimate the USG value with ambient temperatures greater than 68°F (20 C); error increases as temperature increases (Stockham and Scott 2008).

Often, temperature-compensated refractometers provide scales that are calibrated for normal human urine, but veterinary refractometers calibrated for assessment of canine and feline urine are available. The USG difference between dogs and humans is less pronounced than for cats; using the calibration scale for dogs overestimates cat USG (Stockham and Scott 2008). Of the veterinary refractometer models, two provide a distinct scale for determination of USG in cats (VETMED Refractometer, Misco Refractometer, Cleveland, OH; VET 360, Leica Microsystems, Buffalo, NY) (George 2001) (Table 3.1). Quality control and calibration methods for refractometers are discussed in Chapter 8.

Refractometry test limitations
Urine specimens with a specific gravity reading greater than the upper limit obtained by refractometry can be diluted with water and retested, although the degree of concentration may be irrelevant (Table 3.2).

Dry reagent strips

Dipstick methods for specific gravity assessment are inaccurate for veterinary specimens and not recommended, although detailed information regarding the dipstick test methodology can be found in Chapter 4.

Table 3.1 Procedure for determining urine specific gravity by refractometer

Title	Specific gravity procedure
Purpose	The concentrating and diluting function of the kidney is reflected in the solute concentration of the urine measured by specific gravity. Specific gravity is defined as the ratio of the weight of a volume of urine to the weight of the same volume of water. Specific gravity is related to refractive index, which can be measured conveniently with a refractometer.
Specimen	Urine, centrifuged or uncentrifuged
Equipment/reagents/ supplies	Urinalysis Refractometer—Leica Vet 360 Distilled water Kimwipe Disposable pipette
Quality control	Two levels of control are analyzed using the procedure below on a daily basis.
Procedure	1. Lift the cover plate to expose the measuring prism of the refractometer. 2. Place one drop of urine sample on the test plate. 3. Close the cover plate over the prism without delay. 4. To hold the instrument for reading, place finger(s) on cover plate and press gently but firmly. This spreads the sample in a thin, even layer over the prism. Point the refractometer toward a light source. 5. Take the reading at the point where the dividing lines between light and dark field cross the scale. Read the specific gravity from the appropriate scale. There are two scales to read from: the first from the left is for dogs and other large animals; the second is for cats. 6. Document results on the urinalysis report form. 7. Using a few drops of distilled water and a Kimwipe, clean the refractometer by wiping the prism and bottom surfaces of the cover plate.
Results	Results are reported to the third decimal place. Since the result is a ratio, there are no units. Results are recorded onto the urinalysis report form; quality control results are recorded on the quality control spreadsheet.

Sources: Data from Hubbard (1997); McClatchey (1994).

Table 3.2 Calculation for dilution of USG

Procedure for dilution	Add 50 μL of urine sample to 50 μL deionized water. (This is a 1:2 dilution.) Mix well. Read specific gravity (SG) using refractometry.
Calculation	Multiply decimal portion of specific gravity reading by the dilution factor.
Example	Initial refractometer result: >1.050 Result after 1:2 dilution: 1.035 Calculation: 0.035 × 2 Final specific gravity result = 1.070

Source: Data from Strasinger and DiLorenzo (2008).

Table 3.3 Clinical uses for USG

Confirm polyuria

Determine or confirm patient's hydration status

Assess renal function and the kidney's capacity to conserve or excrete water

Allow for estimation of urine loss of protein or other substances (i.e., bilirubin)

Urine volume related to USG

Urine volume, which is also a physical characteristic of urine, is not easily determined in clinical practice due to the necessity of a metabolic cage. Urine volume can be inferred from USG as these are inversely related: low output is associated with concentrated urine while dilute specimens are associated with increased volume.

Expected USG

Adequate USG is >1.030 and >1.035 in dogs and cats, respectively, but maximum concentrating ability is even greater. USG varies in normal animals depending on water intake and hydration status: dogs (1.015–1.045) and cats (1.035–1.065) (Osborne and Stevens 1999; Stockham and Scott 2008; Wamsley and Alleman 2007). To properly assess a patient's ability to dilute or concentrate urine, knowledge of hydration status by physical exam and/or biochemical evaluation and awareness of current medications is necessary. Clinical use and interpretation of USG are found in Tables 3.3 and 3.4, respectively.

Renal ability to concentrate urine persists until greater than two-thirds of functioning nephrons are lost, and so adequate USG may not always reflect kidney health. In some cats with renal disease, renal concentrating ability can

Table 3.4 Interpretation of USG

USG	Significance	Interpretation

>1.030 (dog)
>1.035 (cat)
	Urine is more concentrated than the glomerular ultrafiltrate.
	    Adequate renal function
	    Dehydration or hypoperfusion should be considered in a dehydrated patient
		Hypersthenuria
		Adequately concentrated urine

1.013–1.029 (dog)
1.013–1.034 (cat)
	Urine is more concentrated than the glomerular ultrafiltrate.
	    Renal function may be normal–USG in dogs is more variable.
	    If patient is dehydrated or azotemic, renal insufficiency or extra-renal impairment of concentrating ability is likely (Table 3.5).
		Hypersthenuria
		Moderately concentrated urine

1.008–1.012	Urine, plasma and glomerular ultrafiltrate osmolality are similar.
	    Potentially normal renal function– reevaluation is warranted.
	    If patient is dehydrated or azotemic, renal failure is likely.
		Isosthenuria

<1.008	Urine is more dilute than the glomerular ultrafiltrate.
	    Renal tubules are able to reabsorb solutes from tubular fluid.
	    Consider extrarenal causes of inadequate urine concentration (osmotic diuresis, decreased medullary concentration gradient, etc.) (Table 3.5).
		Hyposthenuria
		Dilute urine

Source: Data from Gregory (2003); Stockham and Scott (2008); Watson (1998).

persist even when biochemical measures of renal disease are present (Hardy and Osborne 1979; Osborne et al. 1995). Causes of inadequate urine concentrating ability can be found in Table 3.5.

Osmolality

Osmolality is the concentration of solutes in a solution and provides a measure of urine concentration (Stockham and Scott 2008; Watson 1998). Urine osmolality can be approximated from the refractive index of urine and the USG, but osmometry, specifically freezing point osmometry, provides a more accurate measure and is less influenced by solution properties. Laboratory analysis of osmolality is impractical for clinical practice but is available

Table 3.5 Causes of inadequate urine concentration

Renal failure

Prolonged diuresis

Lack of ADH (central diabetes insipidus)

Osmotic diuresis (glucosuria; treatment with mannitol)

Excess glucocorticoids (treatment with glucocorticoids, hyperadrenocorticism)

Use of loop diuretics (alters sodium and chloride transport in the loop of Henle)

Decreased renal medullary concentration gradient leading to medullary washout
  Hyponatremia or hypochloremia
  Low urea (hepatic failure or portosystemic shunt)

Lack of response by distal renal tubules to ADH (nephrogenic diabetes insipidus)
  e.g., canine pyometra, hypercalcemia, hyperkalemia

from referral laboratories. Specific measurement of urine osmolality is infrequently necessary in clinical cases.

Urine color

Normal urine color is yellow, but can vary from pale to dark yellow or amber. Pale yellow urine often corresponds to more dilute urine, and dark yellow urine typically corresponds to more concentrated urine. The yellow color is due to the presence of urochromes and urobilin in the urine; both are by-products of normal metabolic processes (Osborne and Stevens 1999). Another pigment, uroerythrin, contributes pink color to human urine specimens, but its presence is not described in veterinary samples.

   In the laboratory, urine samples should be examined for color through a clear container utilizing a good light source and a white background. Technical variation can be minimized by sample comparison to standardized color charts.

Normal and abnormal urine color

The term pigmenturia is generally used to describe abnormal urine color, which can vary from colorless to black. Variations may be due to normal metabolic functions, physical exertion, drug administration, or pathological conditions, although urine color is often used as an indicator of hydration status. Table 3.6 lists differentials for various types of pigmenturia. As one color can have more than one potential cause, chemical analysis and microscopic evaluation are necessary to identify the cause of pigmenturia (Figure 3.2).

Chapter 3

Table 3.6 Laboratory correlations to urine color

Urine color	Differentials
Colorless or pale yellow	Dilute, poorly concentrated urine
Dark yellow to orange	Concentrated urine (dark yellow) Bilirubinuria (orange to orange-brown)
Yellow green	Photo-oxidation of bilirubin in bilirubinuria Biliverdin
Yellow-brown to brown	Bilirubinuria
Red	Hematuria Hemoglobinuria
Red-brown	Hematuria Hemoglobinuria Myoglobinuria Methemoglobin
Brown to black	Methemoglobin Oxyglobin administration Metronidazole administration[a]
Deep red to port wine	Porphyrins
Blue green[a]	Methocarbamol (Robaxin) Methylene blue Amitriptyline (Elavil)

[a] Reported in humans.
Sources: Data from Ben-Ezra et al. (2007); Gregory (2003); Stockham and Scott (2008).

Clarity

Clarity pertains to the transparency or turbidity of a urine specimen. Visual examination of a well-mixed urine sample should be evaluated through a clear specimen container, and results should be reported using consistent terms. Reporting guidelines can be found in Table 3.7. Freshly voided normal urine is usually clear; clear urine specimens, however, may contain chemical abnormalities not detected through visual assessment. Following storage or refrigeration, urine can become cloudy due to the precipitation of salts (Albasan et al. 2003; Stockham and Scott 2008), amorphous phosphates, carbonates, and urates; upon warming the specimen to room temperature, these are expected to dissolve. Microscopic evaluation should always be performed on any urine sample with diminished clarity.

Odor

Characterizing urine odor is not a physical property typically reported as a part of urinalysis, but certain disease processes and drug metabolites can alter urine odor and impact interpretation of test results. A pronounced ammonia odor results from aged urine specimens or can be the result of

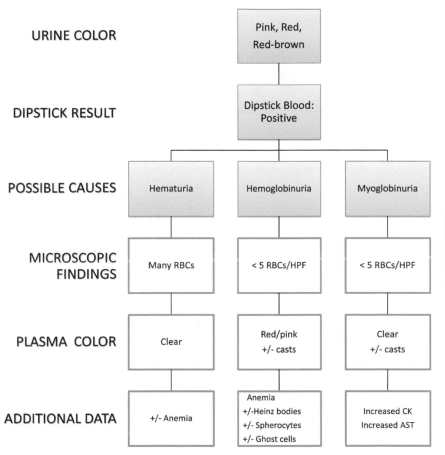

Figure 3.2 Differential diagnosis of red color urine.
RBC, red blood cell; HPF, high power field; CK, creatine kinase; AST, aspartate transaminase.

Table 3.7 Correlation to urine clarity

Urine transparency	Description	Possible clinical correlations
Clear	No turbidity No visible particles Newsprint visible through specimen	Normal Inadequately concentrated urine
Hazy, cloudy, turbid	No visible particles although clarity is increasingly obscured	Mucus Cellular elements Crystalluria
Milky	White, turbid specimen	Pyuria Lipiduria Chyluria (rare)
Flocculent	Many large particles observed	Precipitation of crystals Fecal contamination

bacterial urease. An acetone smell to the urine suggests ketonemia. Administration of various drugs could also result in an altered urine odor. Distinctive chemical smells may indicate contamination via specimen preservatives, strong disinfectants, or skin cleansers.

References

Albasan H, Lulich JP, Osborne CA, Lekcharoensuk C, Ulrich LK, Carpenter KA. 2003. Effects of storage time and temperature on pH, specific gravity, and crystal formation in urine samples from dogs and cats. *Journal of the American Veterinary Medical Association* **222**(2): 176-9.

Ben-Ezra J, Zhao S, McPherson R. 2007. Basic examination of urine. In *Henry's Clinical Diagnosis and Management by Laboratory Methods*, 21st ed. McPherson RA, Pincus MR, eds., pp. 393-409. Philadelphia: Saunders Elsevier.

Free HM. 1987. *Modern Urine Chemistry*. Elkhart, IN: Miles Laboratories.

George JW. 2001. The usefulness and limitations of hand-held refractometers in veterinary laboratory medicine: an historical and technical review. *Veterinary Clinical Pathology* **30**(4): 201-10.

Goldberg HE. 1997. *Principles of Refractometry*. Buffalo, NY: Leica.

Gregory CR. 2003. Urinary system. In *Duncan & Prasse's Veterinary Laboratory Medicine Clinical Pathology*, 4th ed. Latimer KS, Mahaffey EA, Prasse KW, eds., pp. 231-59. Ames, IA: Iowa State Press.

Hardy RM, Osborne CA. 1979. Water deprivation test in the dog: maximal normal values. *Journal of the American Veterinary Medical Association* **174**: 479-83.

Hubbard JD. 1997. *A Concise Review of Clinical Laboratory Science*. Philadelphia: Lippincott Williams & Wilkins.

McClatchey KD. 1994. *Clinical Laboratory Medicine*, 1st ed. Philadelphia: Lippincott Williams & Wilkins.

Osborne CA, Stevens JB. 1999. *Urinalysis: A Clinical Guide to Compassionate Patient Care*. Shawnee Mission, KS: Bayer Corporation.

Osborne CA, Stevens JB, Lulich JD et al. 1995. A clinician's analysis of urinalysis. In *Canine and Feline Nephrology and Urology*. : Osborne CA, Finco DR, eds., pp. 136-205. Baltimore, MD: Williams and Wilkins.

Stockham SL, Scott MA. 2008. Urinary system. In *Fundamentals of Veterinary Clinical Pathology*, 2nd ed. Stockham SL, Scott MA, eds., pp. 415-94. Ames, IA: Blackwell Publishing.

Strasinger SK, DiLorenzo MS. 2008. Physical examination of urine. In *Urinalysis and Body Fluids*, 5th ed. Strasinger SK, DiLorenzo MS, eds., pp. 41-51. Philadelphia: FA Davis Company.

Wamsley H, Alleman R. 2007. Complete urinalysis. In *BSAVA Manual of Canine and Feline Nephrology and Urology*, 2nd ed. Elliott J., Grauer GF, eds., pp. 87-104. Gloucester: British Small Animal Veterinary Association.

Watson ADJ. 1998. Urine specific gravity in practice. *Australian Veterinary Journal* **76**(6): 392-98.

Chapter 4
Routine Urinalysis: Chemical Analysis

Laboratory methods leading to the development of "dip and read" dry reagent systems were invented in the 1940s and revolutionized urinalysis testing during the next two decades. Present-day, dry reagent test strips, or dipsticks, are reliable, easy to use, and provide a rapid means of performing chemical analysis of urine.

Dipsticks consist of chemically impregnated test pads attached to a plastic strip (Figure 4.1). When the test pad is immersed in urine, a color-producing chemical reaction occurs. The color intensity can be examined visually and compared to a manufacturer-supplied chart or interpreted by instrumentation exclusively designed to read test strips. Test results are primarily semi-quantitative although some tests can be estimated in milligrams per deciliter. Laboratory guidelines for dry reagent strips can be found in Table 4.1.

Dry reagent strips are available in a variety of test configurations from different manufacturers, and the brand and format utilized is based on clinical preference. The three major brands are manufactured under the trade names Chemstrip® (Roche Diagnostic Corporation Indianapolis, IN), Idexx UA™ (Idexx Laboratories, Westbrook, ME), and Multistix® (Siemens Healthcare Diagnostics, Tarrytown, NY). The user is advised to closely scrutinize packet inserts and color charts as these are not interchangeable between manufacturers.

This chapter reviews the clinical significance and test methodology of individual dipstick chemistry tests as well as interfering substances that can affect result interpretation. Variations between manufacturers are highlighted when differences exist.

pH

Clinical significance

In most species during health, various acids are produced as a result of normal metabolism and are excreted, in part, by the kidneys. Urine pH is a

Practical Veterinary Urinalysis, First Edition. Carolyn Sink, Nicole Weinstein.
© 2012 John Wiley & Sons, Inc. Published 2012 by John Wiley & Sons, Inc.

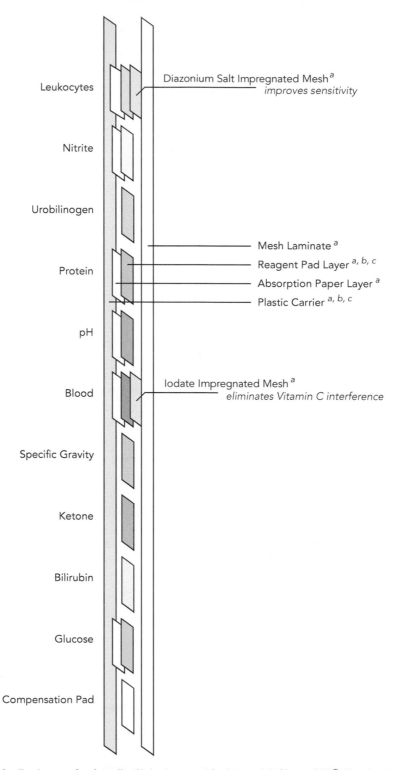

Leukocytes — Diazonium Salt Impregnated Mesh[a]
improves sensitivity

Nitrite

Urobilinogen

Mesh Laminate [a]
Reagent Pad Layer [a, b, c]
Protein — Absorption Paper Layer [a]
Plastic Carrier [a, b, c]

pH

Blood — Iodate Impregnated Mesh [a]
eliminates Vitamin C interference

Specific Gravity

Ketone

Bilirubin

Glucose

Compensation Pad

Figure 4.1 Features of urine dipsticks by manufacturer: (a) Chemstrip® (Roche Diagnostic Corporation Indianapolis, IN), (b) Idexx UA™ (Idexx Laboratories Westbrook, ME), and (c) Multistix® (Siemens Healthcare Diagnostics, Tarrytown, NY).
Sources: Chemstrip 10 MD Product Insert (2007); Idexx UA Strips Product Insert (2002); Multistix Product Insert (2009).

Table 4.1 Laboratory guidelines for dry reagent strips

Storage of reagent strips

Keep container securely sealed.
Do not remove desiccant packet from container.
Protect from temperature extremes and excessive moisture.

Care of reagent strips

Consult packet insert and color chart for changes in procedure, color reactivity or interferences.
Do not use past expiration date.
Remove strip from container immediately prior to use.
Verify test pads are not discolored as this may indicate loss of reactivity.
Do not touch test pads with hands.
Do not perform testing in the presence of alkaline fumes or volatile acids.

Test procedure

Analyze fresh, well-mixed urine sample. If refrigerated, allow specimen to warm to room temperature prior to testing.
Completely submerge test strip briefly (no longer than 1 second) into the urine sample.
Drain excess urine from the test strip by withdrawing the strip against the rim of the container or blot the edge of the strip on absorbent paper. Do not allow test pad reagents to leach.
Compare test pad color reactions to the manufacturer's color chart at specified time intervals. Use a good light source.
Perform confirmatory tests as necessary.

Interpretation of results

Understand the significance of each test result.
Be familiar with the sensitivity, specificity, and sources of error for each test on the reagent strip.
Relate physical, chemical, and microscopic findings.

Sources: Data from Ben-Ezra et al. (2007); Strasinger and DiLorenzo (2008).

result of total body acid–base balance and is influenced by diet, diurnal variation, and disease state.

Precise urine pH measurement is best performed using a pH meter (Johnson et al. 2007), but this method is impractical for clinical use since frequent maintenance and calibration of the device is necessary. Thus, urine pH is routinely obtained using dry chemical reagent strips.

Reagent strip methodology

All dry chemical reagent strips utilize an indicator system consisting of methyl red and bromthymol blue; these indicators react specifically with hydrogen ions in the urine sample to produce visible color on the reagent strip pH test pad.

Dynamic range

The test range provided by Chemstrip and Idexx UA reagent strips is 5–9; readings increment by 1 pH unit. Results obtained by Multistix test strips increment by 0.5 pH unit and range from 5.0 to 8.5 when read visually, and from 5.0 to 9.0 when readings are obtained from automated readers.

Expected value

The expected value is 6.0–7.5 in dogs and cats.

Interferences

There are no known analytical interferences with dry chemical strip methodology for pH, although preanalytical variables may contribute to aberrant values. Acidic urine is associated with high protein diet and is considered normal in carnivores (Table 4.2).

Confirmatory testing

While confirmation of urine pH obtained by dry chemical analysis is rarely indicated, a pH meter, litmus paper strips, or nitrazine paper can be used to verify an unexpected or extreme value.

Protein

Clinical significance

Normal urine contains little to no detectable protein. The minute amounts of protein sometimes present in urine are attributed to various low molecular weight (LMW) plasma proteins (less than 40–60 kD), proteins secreted by renal tubular epithelial cells (i.e. Tamm Horsfall protein), proteins from the distal urogenital tract in free catch or catheterized samples, and usually nondetectable amounts of albumin. Albumin, a medium molecular weight protein (65–70 kD), is mostly absent from normal urine due to selective glomerular filtration. Proximal renal tubular epithelial cells reabsorb the normal small amount of protein passing through the glomerulus and entering into the ultrafiltrate. The capacity of the proximal tubular cells to reabsorb this protein can be saturated or overwhelmed. The amount and type(s) of protein, glomerular filtration, and reabsorptive machinery of the proximal tubular epithelial cells determine final urine protein levels (Stockham and Scott 2008).

Both albumin and non-albumin proteins may be detected during routine urinalysis and/or acid precipitation (confirmatory) methods (Osborne and Stevens 1999; Stockham and Scott 2008; Strasinger and DiLorenzo 2008). Protein is more likely to be detected by a urine dipstick when present in concentrated urine specimens.

Table 4.2 Causes of varied urine pH

Acidic urine
  High protein diet (meat or milk-based)
  Increased protein catabolism
    Starvation
    Corticosteroids
    Muscle wasting
  Metabolic acidosis
    Uremia (renal failure)
    Ethylene glycol toxicosis
    Lactate (severe tissue hypoperfusion)
    Ketones (diabetic ketosis or ketoacidosis)
  Paradoxical aciduria
    Gastric outflow obstruction causing vomiting and dehydration
    (see concurrent hypochloremia, metabolic alkalosis, hypokalemia)
  Hypokalemia
  Bacterial infection (*E. coli* UTI)
  Renal tubular acidosis
    Proximal (if bicarbonate is depleted)
  Diuretics
    Furosemide
  Urinary acidifiers
    Methionine
    Ammonium chloride
    Ascorbic acid (debatable)
Alkaline urine
  Aged urine specimen
    Degradation of urea and loss of CO_2
  Vegetable-based diet
  Metabolic alkalosis +/− respiratory alkalosis
  UTIs due to urease-containing bacteria (i.e., *Proteus, Staphylococcus*)
  Therapeutic agents
    Acetazolamide
    Potassium citrate
    Sodium bicarbonate
  Post-prandial alkaline tide (urine collected 1 hour after a meal)
  Renal tubular acidosis
    Distal (pH may or may not be alkaline)
    Proximal (early)

Sources: Data from Gregory (2003); Osborne and Stevens (1999); Stockham and Scott (2008).

Causes of proteinuria

Causes of proteinuria can be classified based on origin of the protein and can be a result of prerenal or overflow proteinuria, renal and postrenal causes, and tubular secretion of protein.

Prerenal proteinuria

Prerenal or overflow proteinuria is caused by conditions that increase plasma protein levels prior to entering the kidney: myoglobin from muscle injury, hemoglobin from intravascular hemolysis (IVH), Bence-Jones proteins (immunoglobulin light chains) either from plasma cell neoplasia or certain infections, and acute phase reactants increased due to inflammation and infection. Prerenal proteinuria is not expected to directly result in hypoalbuminemia. Some of these proteins and disease processes, however, may result in renal injury.

Renal proteinuria

This category of proteinuria is associated with true renal disease and may be caused by glomerular disease, tubular disease, a combination of glomerular and tubular disease, or, less often, renal interstitial disease. Renal proteinuria can be transient (i.e. a result of fever) or persistent; persistent types of proteinuria are of the greatest clinical concern (Lees et al. 2005; Osborne and Stevens 1999; Strasinger and DiLorenzo 2008).

Glomerular damage

Damage to the glomerular filtration barrier increases glomerular permeability and so increases the amount of plasma proteins, including albumin, in the urine. Causes of glomerular proteinuria are numerous and include both acquired and inherited causes with prognosis depending on exact etiology (Littman 2011). Glomerular proteinuria typically causes a greater amount of albumin loss, which can result in hypoalbuminemia and other complications.

Tubular damage

As mentioned above, proximal renal tubular epithelial cells normally reabsorb and process small amounts of filtered LMW proteins and albumin, when present. When renal tubules are damaged or diseased, they are unable to reabsorb either LMW protein or albumin resulting in proteinuria. Depending on the etiology of the disease or injury, other signs of renal disease may be apparent as well (i.e. azotemia, inadequately concentrated urine, casts). Inherited diseases should be suspected in a younger patient with proteinuria. Acquired tubular proteinuria may result from patients with acute renal disease due to infectious diseases, hypoxia, hypotension, or toxic insults

Chapter 4

(Osborne and Stevens 1999; Stockham and Scott 2008; Strasinger and DiLorenzo 2008).

Postrenal proteinuria

Protein can be added to urine at any point after entering the renal pelvis (i.e. ureter, urinary bladder, or urethra) or from extraurinary sources (genital tract) (Lees 2005). Sources include inflammation due to bacterial or fungal infections, idiopathic inflammatory processes, blood from trauma, neoplasia, or proestrus, prostatic fluid and large amounts of spermatozoa (Osborne and Stevens 1999; Prober et al. 2010; Stockham and Scott 2008; Strasinger and DiLorenzo 2008).

Tubular secretion

Renal epithelial cells in the distal tubule can produce and secrete small amounts of protein which may be detected in concentrated urine samples. The presence of these proteins is considered normal and does not reflect renal disease.

Reagent strip methodology

The protein test methodology used for dry reagent strips is based on the ability of protein to alter an acid-base indicator while the pH of the test medium remains unchanged. In this protein "error of pH indicators" methodology, the acid-base indicator donates hydrogen ions to most proteins present in the urine sample, although it more readily donates hydrogen ions to albumin since it contains more amino groups to accept hydrogen ions (Strasinger and DiLorenzo 2008). The exchange of hydrogen ions results in activation of the chromogen and produces visible color change on the test pad.

Expected value: Negative

Detection of less than 30 mg/dL of protein can be a normal finding in a single well-concentrated specimen (specific gravity greater than 1.025), while persistent proteinuria warrants investigation (Stockham and Scott 2008). Urine protein results should be interpreted in association with specific gravity. Any positive protein result found in dilute urine should be investigated further (Wamsley and Alleman 2007). Chapter 6, "Proteinuria," provides supplementary information on interpretation and additional testing.

Dynamic range

Negative to 3+ (500 mg/dL) Chemstrip
Negative to 3+ (500 mg/dL) Idexx UA
Negative to 4+ (>2000 mg/dL) Multistix

Chapter 4

Table 4.3   Differentials and interferences for urine protein (dipstick)

Positive reaction
  Albumin
  Myoglobin
  Hemoglobin
  Immunoglobulins
  Bence-Jones proteins
  Acute phase proteins
  Mucoproteins
    Tamm-Horsfall (uromodulin) in dogs
    Cauxin in cats

False positive
  Highly alkaline urine
  Chlorhexidine (skin cleanser)
  Blood substitutes (Oxyglobin®)
  Highly pigmented urine samples
  Phenazopyridine (urinary tract analgesic)
  Disinfectants (quaternary ammonium compounds)
  Prolonged immersion of urine sample
    Loss of reagents from dipstick
  Highly buffered urine samples (Multistix®)
    Runover between the pH and adjacent protein test pad

Negative reaction
  Presence of nonalbumin proteins (these may or may not be detected)
  Albumin concentrations of <30 mg/dL (includes microalbuminuria)
  Low pH (false negative)

Sources: Data from Gregory (2003); Miyazaki et al. (2003); Stockham and Scott (2008); Strasinger and DiLorenzo (2008); Wamsley and Alleman (2007).

Chapter 4

Interferences

Refer to Table 4.3.

Confirmatory testing

Sulfosalicylic acid method

The sulfosalicylic acid (SSA) method is a cold precipitation test: when acid is mixed with protein, the protein immediately precipitates, resulting in visual turbidity within the sample. The SSA test screens for all types of protein, but any substance that is precipitated by acid can cause a false-positive reaction (Table 4.3). Precipitate from radiographic dyes can mimic a positive reaction especially when the urine–SSA mixture is left at room temperature.

Table 4.4 Differentials and interferences for SSA testing

Positive reaction
  Presence of:
    Albumin
    Hemoglobin
    Myoglobin
    Globulin
    Bence-Jones proteins
    Glycoproteins
      Tamm-Horsfall (uromodulin) in dogs
      Cauxin in cats

False positive
  Antibiotics:
    Penicillins
    Cephalosporin
    Sulfonamides
  Radiographic contrast agents*
  Uncentrifuged urine sample
  Thymol (urine preservative)
  Tolbutamide (oral hypoglycemic agent)

False negative
  Highly alkaline urine specimen
    Increased pH interferes with acid precipitation

Sources: Data from Gregory (2003); Miyazaki et al. (2003); Osborne and Stevens (1999); Stockham and Scott (2008).

Chapter 4

To perform the SSA test, urine supernatant is mixed with an equal part of 5% SSA, and the amount of precipitate is graded negative to 4+. It is important to utilize centrifuged urine as formed elements or extraneous materials found in uncentrifuged urine can cause false-positive results (Table 4.4).

Detection of microalbuminuria

Microalbuminuria is the presence of urinary albumin greater than normal levels but below the detection level of dry reagent strips, typically 1–30 mg/dL. Semiquantitative reagent strip methods were developed to identify microalbuminuria in human patients at risk for renal disease (Futrakul et al. 2009; Strasinger and DiLorenzo 2008). Microalbuminuria assays that employ immunologic methods specific for human albumin or dye binding detection methods have been shown to be of variable utility in dogs and are not recommended for use in cats (Pressler et al. 2002; Welles et al. 2006). Dipsticks used to detect microalbuminuria with species-specific antibodies to albumin demonstrate greater sensitivity and specificity and is useful in both dogs and cats (Lyon et al. 2010). The reader is guided to Chapter 6 for further discussion of microalbuminuria.

Glucose

Clinical significance

Glucose is a relatively small molecule and freely passes through the glomerulus into the ultrafiltrate. In renal proximal tubular cells, glucose is reabsorbed by both active and facilitated glucose transport systems (Lee et al. 2008). Concomitant hyperglycemia does not always accompany glucosuria since glomerular blood flow, tubular reabsorption rate, and urine flow will influence the presence of glucose in the urine. Nonetheless, glucosuria usually occurs during hyperglycemia when the plasma glucose level exceeds the renal glucose threshold level, which varies by species:

- Dogs: 180-220 mg/dL
- Cats: 280-290 mg/dL

(Gregory 2003; Stockham and Scott 2008)

There are many conditions associated with glucosuria listed in Table 4.5.

Reagent strip methodology

Reagent strip methodology is based on a two-step enzymatic process which employs glucose oxidase and peroxidase. In the initial reaction, glucose oxidase catalyzes glucose and produces gluconic acid and hydrogen peroxide. Subsequently, peroxidase catalyzes the reaction of hydrogen peroxide with a chromogen to produce color. Chromogens utilized for this methodology vary by reagent strip manufacturer; as always, appropriate color charts must be consulted for reaction grading. This reaction is specific for glucose and will not detect reducing substances or other reducing sugars.

Dynamic range

Normal to 1000 mg/dL Chemstrip
Negative to 4+ (1000 mg/dL) Idexx UA
Negative to 4+ (2000 mg/dL or greater) Multistix

Expected value

Normal or negative

Interferences

Refer to Table 4.5.

False positives

Samples obtained from an examination table or floor are most susceptible to contamination by oxidizing agents which may result in false positives (Stockham and Scott 2008).

Table 4.5 Differentials and interferences for glucosuria

Positive result
  Concurrent hyperglycemia
  Mechanism: Plasma glucose level exceeds tubular reabsorption capacity
    Causes:
      Diabetes mellitus
      Glucocorticoids–exogenous or endogenous (uncommon)
      Excitement in cats (typically transient)
      Intravenous glucose supplementation
      +/– Acute pancreatitis
      +/– Pheochromocytoma
      +/– Ethylene glycol intoxication
  Normal plasma glucose (Euglycemia)
  Mechanism: Decreased tubular reabsorption of glucose
    Acquired causes:
      Renal tubular injury, toxicosis, or necrosis of the proximal renal
      tubular epithelial cells
        Nephrotoxic drugs (aminoglycosides, amphotericin B, NSAIDs,
        high dose amoxicillin)
        Severe hypoxemia, hypovolemia or hypotension
        Infectious agents
        Neoplasia
    Inherited/congenital causes:
      Fanconi-like syndrome syndrome or primary renal glucosuria (e.g.,
      Basenji, Norwegian elkhound, Shetland sheepdog)

False positive
  Oxidizing agents
    Hydrogen peroxide
    Hypochlorite (chlorine bleach)

False negative
  Marked bilirubinuria
  Formalin (used as a urine preservative)
  Refrigerated specimens not warmed to room temperature prior to
  testing
  +/– Ketonuria in samples with low levels of glucosuria
  +/– Ascorbic acid (endogenous or exogenous)

Sources: Data from Gregory (2003); Osborne and Stevens (1999); Stockham and Scott (2008); Wamsley and Alleman (2007).

Chapter 4

False negatives

False-negative results are due to substances that interfere with the enzymatic reactions of the dry reagent test and prevent oxidation of the chromogen. Most manufacturers have eliminated the interference from a high specific gravity, ascorbic acid, or moderate levels of ketonuria (40 mg/dL; Wamsley and Alleman 2007).

Confirmatory testing

Reducing substances

Copper reduction tests are utilized in human medicine to screen pediatric patients for reducing substances in the urine, specifically galactose, although other sugars will react (i.e. glucose, fructose, and lactose). In veterinary medicine, copper reduction tests can be used to verify a questionable reagent strip reaction in samples demonstrating significant pigmenturia (Stockham and Scott 2008).

The test methodology employs copper, which reacts with the reducing substance to produce cuprous (Cu+) oxide and cuprous hydroxide, producing a visible color change. The Benedict copper reduction method is more sensitive to detection of reducing substances in urine than the single tablet Clinitest® copper reduction method.

Ketone

Clinical significance

Ketones are intermediate products of fat metabolism and form secondary to excess lipid mobilization. Energy production, which typically relies on carbohydrate metabolism, is shifted to break down and utilize lipid and free fatty acids instead of carbohydrates. Ketone bodies include acetone, acetoacetic acid, and beta-hydroxybutyric acid (3-hydroxybutyrate), but only acetoacetate and acetone have the chemical structure of ketones. Ketone bodies enter the urine by both glomerular filtration of plasma and by tubular secretion; only acetone has the ability to be reabsorbed after entering the tubular fluid.

Reagent strip methodology

Detection of ketones in the urine is based on the method of Legal: acetoacetic acid reacts with sodium nitroprusside and produces pink to purple color on the reagent pad. The test does not detect beta-hydroxybutyric acid.

Dynamic range

Negative to 3+ Chemstrip
Negative to 3+ (150 mg/dL) Idexx UA
Negative to Large (160 mg/dL) Multistix

Expected value

Negative

Interferences

Refer to Table 4.6.

Confirmatory testing

Acetest®

Acetest Reagent Tablets (Bayer Corporation, Elkhart, IN) utilizes the same methodology as the strip method, but lactose is added to enhance color differentiation. This method can be employed for samples other than urine,

Table 4.6 Differentials and interferences for ketonuria

Positive
  Ketosis
    Lactation
    Diabetes mellitus
    Prolonged anorexia
    Starvation (especially young animals)
    Extreme exercise (i.e., endurance race)
  Dietary
    Low carbohydrate (higher in fat, protein)
  Hypoglycemia
    Insulinoma
    Sepsis

False positive
  Pigmenturia (Red)
    Hematuria
    Hemoglobinuria
    Prior diagnostic procedures with bromosulphophthalein dye
  Levodopa metabolites (uncommon)
  Highly concentrated, acidic urine (trace reactions)
  Compounds with sulfhydryl groups (i.e., captopril, cystine)

False negative
  Presence of beta hydroxybutyrate
    Beta hydroxybutyrate not detected by reagent strips
  Aged urine specimen
    Acetone is volatized
  Prolonged exposure of reagent pad to moisture
  Bacteriuria
    Acetoacetic acid broken down by bacteria

Sources: Data from Gregory (2003); Osborne and Stevens (1999); Stockham and Scott (2008); Wamsley and Alleman (2007).

Chapter 4

including serum and body fluids. Acetest Reagent Tablets detect from 5 to 80-100 mg/dL of acetoacetic acid (Acetest packet insert).

Blood

Clinical significance

A positive dipstick reaction for blood can result from hematuria, hemoglobinuria, or myoglobinuria; the presence of any of these substances in urine is an abnormal finding. It is important to differentiate between these three causes, given the very different etiologies. Hematuria can be macroscopic or microscopic and is due to the presence of intact red blood cells (RBCs); a minimum number of 5-20 RBCs/µL is needed to produce a positive heme reaction (Stockham and Scott 2008). Hematuria can result from bleeding anywhere within the urinary tract and should be verified with microscopic evaluation. Hemoglobinuria results from the destruction of RBCs within blood vessels (IVH). Severe muscle injury (rhabdomyolysis) can cause myoglobinuria. Urine containing intact erythrocytes or hemoglobin tends to be red-tinged in color while urine containing myoglobin is often red-brown or brown in color (Archer 2005; Stockham and Scott 2008; Strasinger and DiLorenzo 2008).

Reagent strip methodology

This test detects the presence of RBCs, free hemoglobin, and myoglobin in urine. The methodology is based on the pseudoperoxidase activity of hemoglobin or myoglobin. On the reagent test pad, peroxide and a chromogen produce a visible hue when catalyzed by hemoglobin or myoglobin. Two color patterns may distinguish between hematuria or hemoglobinuria/myoglobinuria:

(1) An isolated reaction producing a speckled pattern ranging from sparse to dense indicates intact RBCs. This pattern results from intact RBCs making contact with the reagent pad, which lyses the cells, and free hemoglobin is released.
(2) Uniform color is produced when free hemoglobin or myoglobin is detected.

Reagent strips can detect hemoglobin concentrations associated with as few as 5 RBCs/µL. Care should be taken when correlating the dry chemical results with the microscopic values for red cells since the absorbent pad examines a greater volume of urine (Strasinger and DiLorenzo 2008).

Dynamic range

Negative to about 250 Erythrocytes per microliter (Ery/µL) Chemstrip
Negative to 4+ (250 Ery/µL) Idexx UA
Non-Hemolyzed: Negative to Moderate and Hemolyzed: Negative to Large (3+) Multistix

Expected value

Negative

Interferences

Refer to Table 4.7.

False positives

Several substances can result in a false-positive reaction (Table 4.7). Extraurinary sources of hemorrhage should be excluded, especially in intact female dogs.

False negatives

One preanalytic error resulting in a false-negative result is a failure to mix the urine thoroughly prior to analysis. RBCs settle quickly in collection containers, producing a false-negative test strip result (Strasinger and DiLorenzo 2008). Ascorbic acid, a strong reducing agent, can inactivate the hydrogen peroxide in the reagent pad and produce false-negative results. Both Siemens and Roche have modified their test methodology to decrease interference to

Chapter 4

Table 4.7 Interferences for occult blood (dipstick)

False positive
  Oxidizing agents
    Hypochlorite (chlorine bleach)
    Hydrogen peroxide
  Marked bilirubinuria (bilirubin > 64 mg/L)
  Large amounts of bromide or iodide
  Extraurinary hemorrhage
  Contamination by digested hemoglobin (flea dirt)
  +/− Presence of bacterial or leukocyte peroxidases

False negative
  Inadequately mixed urine
  Failure of RBCs to lyse in reagent pad
  Increased USG
  Presence of:
    Formalin (used as a urine preservative)
    Formaldehyde
    Captopril
  +/− Ascorbic acid

Sources: Data from Stockham and Scott (2008); Strasinger and DiLorenzo (2008); Wamsley and Alleman (2007).

only high levels (25 mg/dL) of ascorbic acid (Strasinger and DiLorenzo 2008). Idexx strips demonstrate no interference with ascorbic acid.

Differentiation of positive results

Refer to Table 4.8.

Hematuria

The presence of RBCs in the urine results from urogenital tract hemorrhage and includes both iatrogenic and pathological causes. Urine collection via cystocentesis, catheterization, or manual expression can all result in iatrogenic hemorrhage. Causes of pathological urinary tract hemorrhage include trauma, inflammation, neoplasia, inherited and acquired primary and secondary hemostatic disorders, and idiopathic disorders.

Hemoglobinuria

Following release of hemoglobin (64 kD) into plasma due to IVH, free hemoglobin dimers (32 kD) form and are scavenged by haptoglobin. Haptoglobin recovers the hemoglobin so as to conserve iron and prevent renal tubular injury by hemoglobin. In severe cases of IVH, the haptoglobin recovery

Table 4.8   Differentials for positive occult blood and red/pink urine color

Condition	Urine			Plasma	Additional data
	Color	Dipstick	Microscopic	Color	CBC/Chemistry
Hematuria	Pink, red, brown	+ Blood +/− Protein	Many RBCs	Normal	+/− Anemia
Hemoglobinuria	Pink, red, brown	+ Blood +/− Protein	None to few RBCs Occasional pigmented casts	Pink	Low PCV/Anemia +/− Heinz bodies +/− Spherocytes +/− Ghost cells +/− Hemic parasites
Myoglobinuria	Red, brown	+ Blood +/− Protein	None to few RBCs Occasional brown casts	Normal	↑CK ↑AST

Source: Data from Stockham and Scott (2008); Strasinger and DiLorenzo (2008); Wamsley and Alleman (2007).

system is overwhelmed, and the excess hemoglobin dimers pass through the glomerulus, enter the ultrafiltrate, and are either resorbed by the renal tubules or are excreted into the urine.

Concurrent pink or red-tinged plasma, indicative of hemoglobinemia, supports a diagnosis of hemoglobinuria. Anemia is expected. The presence of Heinz bodies, ghost cells, hemic parasites (i.e. *Mycoplasma* sp., *Babesia* sp.), or spherocytes on a peripheral blood smear would further support hemolysis. Hemoglobinuria can also develop in cases of hematuria and lysis of RBCs within urine that is very alkaline or dilute (urine specific gravity [USG] < 1.015; Stockham and Scott 2008). Plasma should be clear.

Myoglobinuria

Myoglobin is released from myocyte (muscle cell) damage or necrosis; myoglobin (17 kD) is freely filtered by the glomerulus and will be excreted in the urine if not resorbed by renal tubules. Myoglobinuria imparts a brown or red-brown-tinged color to urine. Distinguishing myoglobinuria from hemoglobinuria can be challenging, given the positive heme reaction for both and the similarly colored urine. Plasma color is expected to be clear when myoglobinuria is present as opposed to hemoglobinuria. Previous recommendations for differentiation of myoglobinuria and hemoglobinuria included an ammonium sulfate precipitation test; it is generally considered unreliable, and other clinicopathological measures (i.e. packed cell volume [PCV], CBC findings, blood smear review, biochemical tests) should be consulted (Ben-Ezra et al. 2007; Stockham and Scott 2008; Strasinger and DiLorenzo 2008). In contrast to large animals, especially horses, myoglobinuria is relatively uncommon in small animals, given the smaller relative muscle mass. Biochemical changes that would be seen concurrently with myoglobinuria include increased levels of plasma creatine kinase (CK) and aspartate transaminase (AST); AST can also elevate with hemolysis so CK is preferred for diagnosis of muscle injury. Myoglobinuria is seen with rhabdomyolysis secondary to muscle trauma or ischemia, and following intense exertion or severe convulsions. Myoglobin can, itself, cause renal tubular injury similar to free hemoglobin. This is less common in small animals than in humans or horses (Stockham and Scott 2008).

Bilirubin

Clinical significance

Bilirubin is a normal product of RBC breakdown. Senescent RBCs are phagocytized by macrophages within the spleen and liver. Within macrophages, iron is extracted from the heme ring, ultimately resulting in the formation of bilirubin. Bilirubin bound to albumin (unconjugated or indirect bilirubin) is taken to the liver for conjugation (conjugated or direct bilirubin), excreted into the biliary tree (bile canaliculi and bile ducts), and then excreted into the intestine. Only conjugated bilirubin is water soluble and able to be freely filtered by the glomerulus. Hyperbilirubinemia (conjugated or unconjugated) and bilirubinuria can result from hemolysis as well as obstructive or functional cholestasis (failure to excrete bilirubin into the biliary tree). Bilirubinuria may precede hyperbilirubinemia in animals with a low renal threshold for bilirubin (i.e. the dog).

Reagent strip methodology

In the presence of bilirubin, diazotized dichloroaniline couples with bilirubin and produces color on the reagent pad. A bilirubin concentration of 0.4 mg/dL is considered negative; test methods with lower sensitivity should be employed to detect lower levels. Reagent strip color reactions for bilirubin are often difficult to discern in urine specimens of normal color; atypical urine pigments intensify this challenge. Confirmatory testing is utilized to verify positive or questionable results.

Dynamic range

Negative to 3+ Chemstrip
Negative to 3+ Idexx UA
Negative to 3+ Multistix

Expected value: Negative

Refer to Table 4.9.

Interferences

False positives

Metabolites of the nonsteroidal anti-inflammatory drug (NSAID) Etodolac can result in false-positive bilirubin dipstick reactions. Intestinal bacterial tryptophan metabolism can produce indican, which can also result in a positive bilirubin test.

False negatives

False negatives can occur when bilirubin is converted to a biliverdin or free bilirubin; neither reacts with bilirubin tests employing diazo. Spontaneous oxidation of bilirubin to biliverdin can result from exposure to ultraviolet light and a prolonged processing delay of urine specimens. False negatives are also observed when free bilirubin is present from the hydrolysis of bilirubin diglucuronide (Strasinger and DiLorenzo 2008). Increased levels of either nitrite or greater than 25 mg/dL of ascorbic acid reduces reaction of the test

Table 4.9 Differentials and interferences for bilirubinuria

Positive
  Normal (dogs)
    Concentrated urine samples may contain small amounts of bilirubin (1+ or less)
  Hemolysis (Intra- or extravascular)
  Cholestasis
    Obstructive hepatic or posthepatic lesions
    Functional (sepsis)

False positive
  Etodolac (NSAID)
  Deeply pigmented urine
  Indican (intestinal bacterial metabolite)
  Hemoglobinemia
    Tubular formation of bilirubin from hemoglobin

False negative
  Delayed processing
  Exposure to ultraviolet light
  Presence of:
    Nitrite
    Ascorbic acid (endogenous or exogenous)

Sources: Data from Archer (2005); Stockham and Scott (2008); Strasinger and DiLorenzo (2008).

pad with bilirubin as both combine with the diazonium salt in the test pad and lowers the sensitivity of the test (Strasinger and DiLorenzo 2008).

Confirmatory test

Ictotest®

The Ictotest (Siemens Medical Solutions Diagnostics, Tarrytown, NY) detects levels of bilirubin as low as 0.05 mg/dL (Strasinger and DiLorenzo 2008), making it an ideal confirmatory test for questionable results. The test kit consists of test mats and tablets containing *p*-nitrobenzene diazonium *p*-toluene sulfonate, SSA, sodium carbonate, and boric acid.

Ictotest procedure: Ten drops of urine are added to the cottony side of one test mat; urine is absorbed on the test mat while bilirubin remains on the surface of the mat. One tablet is centered on the absorbed urine, and one drop of water is placed on the tablet. After 5 seconds, a second drop of water is placed on the tablet, both of which spill onto the mat. The reaction should continue for 60 seconds before the tablet is removed and color is evaluated. Blue to purple is positive for bilirubin; any other color is considered a negative reaction. The Ictotest is less prone to interference than dry reagent strip methods and should be employed when detection of bilirubin levels less than 0.40 mg/dL is necessary (Strasinger and DiLorenzo 2008).

Chapter 4

Urobilinogen

Clinical significance

Conjugated bilirubin is delivered to the intestine where most is converted to urobilinogen by intestinal flora and subsequently excreted. Small amounts of urobilinogen are reabsorbed into portal blood and removed by hepatocytes or excreted into the urine. Urine urobilinogen is colorless. A tetrapyrrole metabolite of bilirubin, urobilinogen is unstable and may be oxidized to urobilin in an acid environment. Additionally, urobilinogen may be converted to urobilin when a urine sample is exposed to ultraviolet light, which turns the urine sample green-tinged.

Since urobilinogen test pads are found on most dry reagent strips used in human medicine, urobilinogen is commonly incorporated in veterinary urinalysis studies. In the dog, extreme cases of hemolysis may produce high urobilinogen levels with detection possible approximately 3 days after the onset of hemolysis (Tang et al. 2008). Hemolytic episodes in other species do not consistently produce urobilinogenuria. Most investigators agree that testing for urobilinogen in dog and cat urine is unreliable.

Reagent strip methodology

Based on the Ehrlich reaction, test pads contain a color enhancer and diazonium salt that reacts with urobilinogen to produce a visible pink-red tint. Results are reported in Ehrlich units per deciliter (EU/dL), which equates to approximately 1 mg/dL. Urobilin or porphobilinogen are not detected by this methodology. Multistix reagent strips can detect urobilinogen in concentrations as low as 0.2 EU/dL; however, the absence of urobilinogen cannot be detected on any dry reagent strip. Results up to 1 mg/dL are considered normal, while a result of 2 EU/dL or greater warrants investigation for hemolytic and hepatic disease.

Dynamic range

Normal to 12 mg/dL Chemstrip
Normal to 4+ (12 mg/dL) Idexx UA
Normal to 8 mg/dL Multistix

Expected value

Normal

Interferences

Refer to Table 4.10.

Table 4.10 Differentials and interferences for urobilinogen

Positive
  Insignificant
False positive
  Darkly colored urine
  Sulphonamides (antibiotic)
  Aminobenzoic acid (PABA)
  Phenazopyridine (urinary tract analgesic)
  Any substance that reacts with Ehrlich reagent
  Aminosalicylic acid (derivative of salicylic acid)
False negative
  Urine specimens exposed to sunlight
  Formalin (used as urine preservative)

Sources: Data from Archer (2005); Stockham and Scott (2008); Strasinger and DiLorenzo (2008); Wamsley and Alleman (2007).

Nitrite

Clinical significance

Nitrate is normally present in the urine of humans and is derived from consumption of nitrate-rich meat, vegetables, and drinking water. In the presence of bacteria that contain nitrite reductase (typically gram-negative bacteria), urinary nitrate is converted to nitrite; detection of nitrituria is associated with gram-negative bacteria infections in humans. However, corroborative data have not been observed in other species, and this test result is generally disregarded if performed on a veterinary sample (Archer 2005; Wamsley and Alleman 2007).

Reagent strip methodology

In the presence of nitrite, para-arsanilic acid forms a diazonium compound which couples with 1,2,3,4-tetrahydrobenzo(h)quinolin-3-ol to produce detectable color on the reagent pad. This methodology is specific for nitrite. A positive result suggests the presence of 1,000,000 or more organisms per milliliter.

Dynamic range

Negative or Positive Chemstrip
Negative to 3+ Idexx UA
Negative or Positive Multistix

Expected value

Negative.

Interferences

False positives

False-positive results are observed with dark-colored urine specimens, urines with high specific gravity, or large amounts of ascorbic acid in the urine (Strasinger and DiLorenzo 2008).

False negative

False-negative results are obtained from patients who lack dietary nitrate or from bacteriuric samples not retained in the bladder for enough time to convert nitrate to nitrite (4 hours) (Strasinger and DiLorenzo 2008). Since urine retention time is commonly unmanageable for veterinary patients, this test a poor diagnostic tool (Archer 2005).

Leukocyte esterase

Clinical significance

This reagent strip test was developed for use in human medicine to eliminate technical variation in urine sediment preparation and examination; it identifies pyuria but does not measure the concentration of leukocytes in the urine sample. This parameter is deemed unreliable for veterinary samples (Archer 2005; Holan et al. 1997; Vail et al. 1986).

Reagent strip methodology

This reagent strip methodology is based on the esterase activity of granulocytic leukocytes. When present in the urine, leukocytic esterase catalyzes the hydrolysis of an amino acid ester to indoxyl on the reagent pad. Indoxyl reacts with diazonium salt on the reagent pad to produce visible color.

Esterases are not present in lymphocytes, erythrocytes, bacteria, or renal cells. Most manufacturers have eliminated interference from non-leukocytic esterases, but the manufacturer packet insert should be consulted for further clarification if needed.

Dynamic range

Negative to 2+ Chemstrip
Not present on Idexx UA
Negative to 3+ Multistix

Expected value

Negative.

Interferences

Given this test is unreliable in veterinary species, false positive and negative reactions have minimal relevance.

False positives

In humans, trace and other positive readings should be investigated. Contamination of the urine specimen with vaginal discharge may cause false-positive readings (Strasinger and DiLorenzo 2008).

False negatives

False negatives may be caused by medications (cephalexin, cephalothin, tetracycline, oxalic acid), ascorbic acid, albuminuria, glucosuria, high specific gravity, or darkly colored urine (Strasinger and DiLorenzo 2008).

Specific gravity

Clinical significance

Specific gravity assessed by dry chemical test strips is unreliable for veterinary specimens (Wamsley and Alleman 2007). Suitable for use with human samples, it is standard test included on many dipstick configruations and is therefore included in this discussion.

Reagent strip methodology

When cations are present in the urine sample, protons are released by a complexing agent in the reagent pad. These protons react with the color indicator to produce visible color.

Dynamic range

1.000–1.030 Chemstrip
Not present on Idexx UA
1.000–1.030 Multistix

Expected value

Not recommended for veterinary specimens.

Interferences

As the reagent strip method measures only ionic solutes, interference by large organic molecules is discounted. For this reason, readings using reagent strip methodology may differ from refractometer readings (Strasinger and DiLorenzo 2008).

False positives

False increases in USG by dry chemical analysis may be found with ketonuria or proteinuria (Strasinger and DiLorenzo 2008).

False negatives

False decreases in USG are found in highly buffered alkaline urines due to interference with the bromthymol blue indicator, and manufacturers recommend adding 0.005 to specific gravity readings when the pH is greater than or equal to 6.5. Automated strip readers can be configured to adjust results following this algorithm (Strasinger and DiLorenzo 2008).

References

Acetest® Reagent Tablet Product Insert. 1995. Bayer Corporation, Elkhart, IN.

Archer J. 2005. Urine analysis. In *BSAVA Manual of Canine and Feline Clinical Pathology*, 2nd ed. Villiers E, Blackwood L, eds., pp. 149–55. Gloucester: British Small Animal Veterinary Association.

Ben-Ezra J, Zhao S, McPherson R. 2007. Basic examination of urine. In *Henry's Clinical Diagnosis and Management by Laboratory Methods*, 21st ed. McPherson RA, Pincus MR, eds., pp. 393–409. Philadelphia: Saunders Elsevier.

Chemstrip® 10 MD Product Insert. 2007. Roche Diagnostics, Indianapolis, IN.

Futrakul N, Sridama V, Futrakul P. 2009. Microalbuminuria: a biomarker of renal microvascular disease. *Renal Failure* **31**(2): 140–3.

Gregory CR. 2003. Urinary system. In *Duncan & Prasse's Veterinary Laboratory Medicine Clinical Pathology*, 4th ed. Latimer KS, Mahaffe EA, Prasse KW, eds., pp. 231–59. Ames, IA: Iowa State Press.

Holan KM, Kruger JM, Gibbons SM, Swenson CL. 1997. Clinical evaluation of a leukocyte esterase test-strip for detection of feline pyuria. *Veterinary Clinical Pathology* **26**(3): 126–31.

Idexx UA™ Strips Product Insert. 2002. Idexx Laboratories, Westbrook, ME.

Johnson KY, Lulich JP, Osborne CA. 2007. Evaluation of the reproducibility and accuracy of pH-determining devices used to measure pH in dogs. *Journal of the American Veterinary Association* **230**(3): 364–9.

Lee YJ, Lee YJ, Han HJ. 2008. Regulatory mechanisms of Na(+)/glucose cotransporters in renal proximal tubule cells. *Kidney International* **73**(3): 361–2.

Lees GE, Brown SA, Elliott J et al. 2005. Assessment and management of proteinuria in dogs and cats: ACVIM Forum Consensus Statement (small animal). *Journal of Veterinary Internal Medicine* **19**: 377–85.

Littman MP. 2011. Protein-losing nephropathy in small animals. *The Veterinary Clinics of North America. Small Animal Practice* **41**(1): 31–62.

Lyon SD, Sanderson MW, Vaden SL, Lappin MR, Jenese WA, Grauer GF. 2010. Comparison of urine dipstick, sulfosalicylic acid, urine protein-to-creatinine ratio, and species-specific ELISA methods for detection of albumin in urine samples of cats and dogs. *Journal of the American Veterinary Association* **236**(8): 874-9.

Miyazaki M, Kamiie K, Soeta S, Taira H, Yamashita T. 2003. Molecular cloning and characterization of a novel carboxylesterase-like protein that is physiologically present at high concentrations in the urine of domestic cats (*Felis catus*). 2003. *The Biochemical Journal* **370**(Pt 1):101-10.

Multistix® Product Insert. 2009. Siemens Healthcare Diagnostics Inc. Tarrytown, NY.

Osborne CA, Stevens JB. 1999. *Urinalysis: A Clinical Guide to Compassionate Patient Care*. Shawnee Mission, KS: Bayer Corporation.

Pressler BM, Vaden SL, Jensen WA, Simpson D. 2002. Detection of canine microalbuminuria using semiquantitative test strips designed for use with human urine. *Veterinary Clinical Pathology* **31**(2): 56-60.

Prober LG, Johnson CA, Olivier NB, Thomas JS. 2010. Effect of semen in urine specimens on urine protein concentration determined by means of dipstick analysis *American Journal of Veterinary Research* **71**: 288-92.

Stockham SL, Scott MA. 2008. Urinary system. In *Fundamentals of Veterinary Clinical Pathology*, 2nd ed. Stockham SL, Scott MA, eds., pp. 415-94. Ames, IA: Blackwell Publishing.

Strasinger SK, DiLorenzo MS. 2008. Chemical examination of urine. In *Urinalysis and Body Fluids*, 5th ed. Strasinger SK, DiLorenzo MS, eds., pp. 53-80. Philadelphia: FA Davis Company.

Tang X, Xia Z, Yu J. 2008. An experimental study of hemolysis induced by onion (*Allium cepa*) poisoning in dogs. *Journal of Veterinary Pharmacology and Therapeutics* **31**(2): 143-9.

Vail DM, Allen TA, Weiser G. 1986. Applicability of leukocyte esterase test strip in detection of canine pyuria. *Journal of the American Veterinary Association* **189**(11): 1451-3.

Wamsley H, Alleman R. 2007. Complete urinalysis. In *BSAVA Manual of Canine and Feline Nephrology and Urology*, 2nd ed. Elliot J, Grauer GF, eds., pp. 87-104. Gloucester: British Small Animal Veterinary Association.

Welles EG, Whatley EM, Hall AS, Wright JC. 2006. Comparison of Multistix PRO dipsticks with other biochemical assays for determining urine protein (UP), urine creatinine (UC) and UP: UC ratio in dogs and cats. *Veterinary Clinical Pathology* **35**(1): 31-6.

Chapter 4

Chapter 5

Routine Urinalysis: Microscopic Elements

Routine urinalysis testing culminates in microscopic evaluation of the urine sediment, which requires a high level of proficiency to assure accurate and relevant results. This chapter contains guidelines for identification and quantification of formed elements. Preparation and analysis of urine sediment is prone to technical variation; protocols developed to standardize these variables are also contained in this chapter (Table 5.1).

Urine sediment preparation

As with all phases of testing, fresh urine is preferred, but appropriate preservation, typically refrigeration, is acceptable, especially when a delay in processing is anticipated. If refrigeration is employed, specimens should be allowed to reach room temperature prior to testing as low temperature may increase formation of amorphous crystals. Formed elements, such as cells and casts, rapidly deteriorate at room temperature. Formed elements also gravitate to the bottom of collection and testing containers, so samples should be well mixed prior to transfer or testing.

Specimen volume

Approximately 5 mL of urine is centrifuged to obtain sediment. Greater amounts (>10 mL) are desirable, but this sample size can be challenging to obtain from some dogs and most cats. Also, centrifugation of larger amounts can be technically challenging given equipment available in general practice. Recording the specific volume of urine centrifuged allows for extrapolation of sediment results per milliliter of urine if desired, although this calculation is not routinely performed (Table 5.2).

Practical Veterinary Urinalysis, First Edition. Carolyn Sink, Nicole Weinstein.
© 2012 John Wiley & Sons, Inc. Published 2012 by John Wiley & Sons, Inc.

Table 5.1 Technical variables affecting microscopic analysis of urine

Delay in testing

Total volume of urine specimen

Method by which the sediment is prepared

Total volume of sediment examined

Quality of equipment used

Timeliness and method of result reporting

Table 5.2 Calculation for reporting elements per milliliter of urine

1. Calculate area of lpf or hpf.
2. Calculate the maximum number of fields in the viewing area.
3. Calculate the number of fields per milliliter of urine tested.
4. Calculate the number of formed elements per milliliter of urine.

Example:

1. Use the field of view specification supplied by the manufacturer and the formulas:
   Area = Π radius² and Diameter = 2 radius
   Manufacturer specification for high power field (hpf) of view = 0.35 mm; thus:
   3.14 × 0.175² = 0.096 mm²
2. Coverslip area (22 mm × 22 mm) = 484 mm²
   484/0.96 = 5040 hpf in entire viewing area
3. 12 mL of urine centrifuged; 0.02 mL sediment examined
   5040 hpf/(0.02 mL × 12 mL) = 21,000 hpf/mL of urine tested
4. For each element observed, multiply the number reported by 21,000:
   5 WBC/hpf × 21,000 hpf/mL = 105,000 WBC/mL

Sources: Data from Free (1986); Strasinger and DiLorenzo (2008).

Centrifugation

Centrifugation speed and duration must be consistent to ensure reliable laboratory results. To concentrate formed elements, specimens should be centrifuged for 5 minutes at a relative centrifugal force (RCF) of 400. Most centrifuge speed settings are in the units of revolutions per minute (RPM), and the appropriate RPM must be calculated using the following formula (Eq. 5.1) by Sink and Feldman (2004):

$$RPM = (\text{square root } [400/28.38R]) \times 1000 \qquad \text{(Eq. 5.1)}$$

where R = radius of centrifuge rotor in inches.

Alternately, conversion nomographs or "speed calculators" can be used to obtain the appropriate RPM setting. Centrifuge rotors may be of swinging bucket or fixed angle, although swinging bucket rotors are advantageous when there is a small amount of precipitate (produces leveled sediment button).

Ideally, samples should be capped prior to centrifugation to prevent bio-hazardous aerosolization. Centrifuge deceleration should not be enhanced by braking as this disrupts the urine sediment.

Sediment preparation

Optimally, a total residual volume of 0.5–1.0 mL of urine and sediment should remain in the tube after the supernatant is aspirated. Pouring off the super-natant is less ideal as overaggressive decanting can compromise sediment consistency. Likewise, vigorous methods utilized to resuspend urine sediment should be avoided; gentle suspension using a pipette or gentle tapping the tip of the tube with the finger is preferred. Complete and thorough resuspen-sion of the sediment is necessary to ensure accurate distribution of the formed elements for microscopic analysis.

Volume of sediment for microscopic analysis

Commonly, a plastic pipette is used to place a small drop of urine on a micro-scope slide; however, using the conventional glass slide method, the recom-mended sediment volume is 20 μL sequestered by a 22 × 22 mm glass coverslip (Strasinger and DiLorenzo 2008). Excessive sample volume must be avoided as heavier formed elements (casts) can flow outside the viewing field. Commercially available slides (KOVA Glasstic® Slide 10, Hycor Biomedi-cal, Garden Grove, CA) containing constant volume chambers allow for even distribution of microscopic elements and minimize associated technical error.

Stain

The decision to stain urine sediment is a matter of personal preference. Supravital staining enhances contrast within the specimen and changes the refractive index of formed elements, thus increasing their overall visibility. The most frequently used supravital stain for urinalysis in veterinary medicine is Sedi-Stain (BD Clay Adams™ Sedi-Stain Concentrated Stain). This is a sta-bilized modification of the Sternheimer-Malbin urinary stain typically used in human medicine and can be used with typical wet mount preparations (Stras-inger and DiLorenzo 2008). Air-dried urine sediments can be stained with a rapid Romanowsky stain such as Diff-Quik (Dade Behring Inc., Newark, NJ).

Examination of urine sediment

Unstained urine sediment is examined under subdued light with the con-denser lowered. The lower condenser position provides the necessary con-trast to identify formed elements in the urine. The condenser should be raised

Table 5.3 Recommended reporting guidelines for microscopic evaluation of urine

| Element | Microscopic power | | Quantification |
	HPF	LPF	
RBC	•		Enumerate range up to 150 cells; if >150 = 4+
WBC	•		Enumerate range up to 150 cells; if >150 = 4+
Epithelial cells	•		Classify type and enumerate range
Casts		•	Classify type and enumerate range
Crystals		•	Rare, Small, Moderate, Large
Bacteria	•		Rare, small, moderate, large
Yeast	•		Rare, small, moderate, large
Parasites	•		Enumerate range up to 150 cells; if >150 = 4+
Mucus	•	•	Rare, small, moderate, large
Other		•	Name and enumerate range

Acceptable range values include 0-2, 3-5, 7-10, and so on.

(to just under the microscope stage), and the light can be increased with stained sediment samples as the stain provides the necessary contrast to visualize structures. Initial focusing on one large formed element provides a point of reference and localizes the plane of view. Subsequent formed elements are often difficult to discern, but this is circumvented through acuity of fine focus. The sediment is examined under low power field (lpf) in order to assess the general composition of the sediment and to visualize larger structures; identification of individual structures is accomplished under high power field (hpf). When using the conventional glass slide method, larger elements tend to flow toward the perimeter of the cover glass necessitating scan of this area. Constant volume chambers do not produce this phenomenon.

Laboratory reporting

Examination of a minimum of 10 fields under both low (10× objective) and high (40× objective) power is necessary to determine sediment content. Ideally, scanning of the entire area covered by the coverslip would be performed on 10× to look for regions with increased density or clumping, which could negatively skew results. Quantification or qualification terminology varies from lab to lab, but must be consistent within one laboratory (see Tables 5.3 and 5.4).

Table 5.4 Procedure for sediment analysis

1. Obtain urine sample. If the sample is refrigerated, allow to warm to room temperature. Mix sample well.

2. Using a pipette, transfer at least 4-5 mL of urine into a clean tube (12 × 75 mm or conical tip centrifuge tube).

3. Centrifuge sample for 5 minutes at 400 × g.

4. If necessary, perform confirmatory tests using supernatant.

5. Decant supernatant, leaving approximately 0.5-1 mL of urine and sediment.

6. Resuspend the sediment by gentle agitation.

7. Using a plastic pipette, transfer a drop of the sediment suspension onto a clean glass slide and cover with a 22 × 2 mm glass coverslip.

8. Lower the microscope condenser to enhance visualization of unstained sediment.

9. Examine the sediment on 10× to evaluate for larger formed elements (i.e. casts and crystals) and to determine overall cellularity. Some parasites can also be identified on low magnification (i.e., microfilaria, *Dioctophyma renale*).

10. Examine the urine sediment on 40× to enumerate RBCs, WBCs, and epithelial cells, and to identify, enumerate, and characterize bacteria, yeast/fungus, parasites, and smaller crystals.

11. Record results.

Chapter 5

Microscopic elements of urine sediment

Red blood cells

In unstained urine sediment, red blood cells (RBCs) are biconcave disks; nuclei are lacking in dogs and cats but are present in some exotic species (Figure 5.1). In fresh urine, RBCs are pale in color, which diminishes with specimen age. In hypersthenuric specimens, RBCs decrease in size due to loss of water; this can lead to crenated or irregular shaped cells (Figure 5.2a,b). In dilute urine (hyposthenuria), RBCs absorb water, swell, and eventually lyse, producing "ghost cells."

Microscopically, RBCs must be distinguished from similarly shaped elements including yeast, lipid droplets, and air bubbles (Figure 5.3a,b). RBCs are most often similarly sized and are smaller than leukocytes. RBCs display a smooth appearance while leukocytes appear more finely granular (Figure 5.4a,b). Differentiation can be achieved by the addition of acetic acid to the sediment; RBCs will lyse while yeast or lipid droplets remain and air bubbles will dissipate. Additionally, non-RBC elements will be inconsistent in size, particularly lipid droplets, which appear spherical and refractile. Yeast is

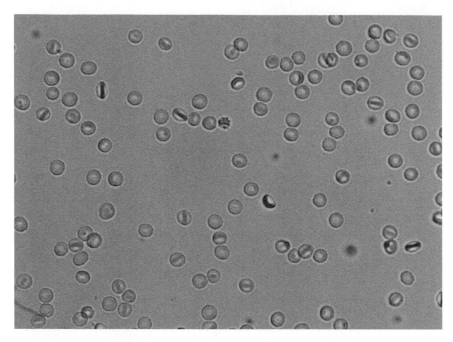

Figure 5.1 Many RBCs, 40×.

often ovoid in shape and exhibits budding. Less than 5 RBCs/hpf is considered normal in dogs and cats. Increased numbers, unrelated to a pathological process, can result from iatrogenic bleeding during cystocentesis.

White blood cells

In contrast to RBCs, white blood cells (WBCs) are approximately 1.5 times larger and contain a round to lobulated nucleus (Figure 5.5). In health and most disease processes, neutrophils predominate although any type of leukocyte may be found. While WBCs are not differentiated in routine urinalysis, knowledge of leukocyte morphology aids in overall classification. Neutrophils contain cytoplasmic granules which swell and exhibit motility when exposed to hypotonic urine, thus explaining the term "glitter cells." Eosinophils are morphologically similar to neutrophils and are only distinguishable if the sediment is stained with Romanowsky-type stains. Small lymphocytes, which possess a high nuclear to cytoplasm ratio, are easily confused with RBCs. The addition of acetic acid to the urine sediment will lyse RBCs and enhance nuclear detail of any WBC, including lymphocytes. Monocytes may be present in low numbers in urine samples containing abundant peripheral blood. Macrophages are the tissue form of monocytes and are uncommonly identified in wet urine sediment preparations, although they may be present in samples from patients with urinary tract

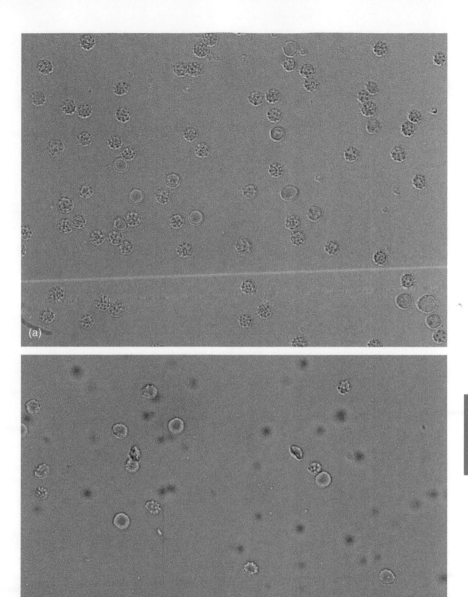

Figure 5.2 (a) Normal and crenated RBCs, 40×; (b) crenated RBCs of varying sizes, 40×.

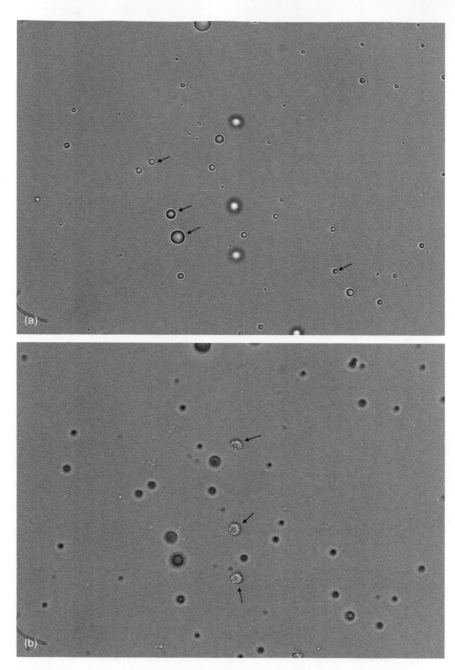

Figure 5.3 RBCs with variably sized lipid droplets: (a) Focused on lipid droplets (arrows), 40×; (b) focused on red blood cells (arrows), 40×.

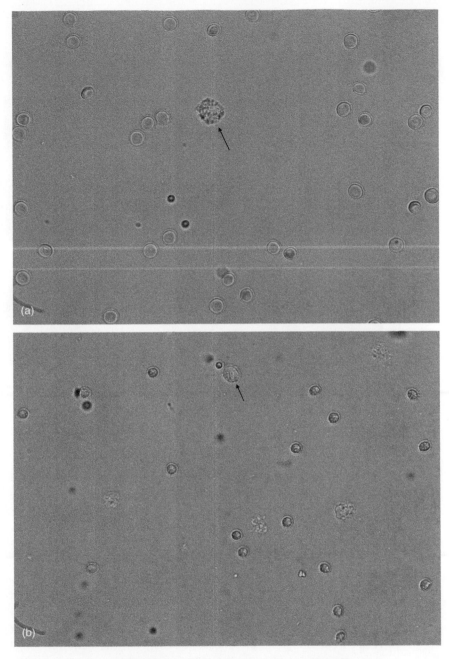

Figure 5.4 (a) and (b) RBCs, WBCs (arrow), lipid droplets, 40×.

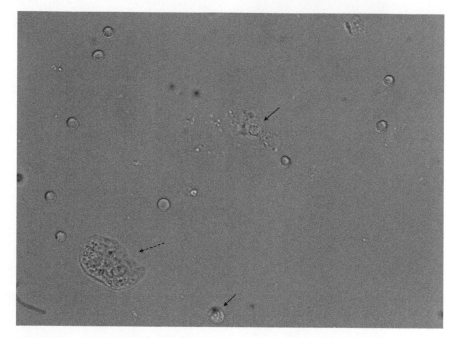

Figure 5.5 RBCs, WBCs (arrows), squamous epithelial cell (dashed arrow), bacteria in background.

Chapter 5

inflammation. Macrophages are usually larger than a neutrophil with an ovoid to lobulated nucleus, and abundant cytoplasm, which may appear vacuolated or contain inclusions. Specimens containing mononuclear cells that cannot be identified should be referred for cytologic evaluation. Greater than 5 WBC/hpf is considered abnormal and suggests underlying urinary tract infection (Figures 5.6a,b-5.11a,b).

Epithelial cells

Epithelial cells are normally found in urine sediment in low numbers and result from sloughing of senescent cells from the genitourinary tract. The three main types of epithelial cells are classified according to their point of origin.

Renal tubular epithelial cells

Renal tubular epithelial cells (RTEs) are uncommonly identified in urine sediment; identification is often hindered by degeneration, which is a result of the transit time from the renal tubule. RTEs vary in morphology depending on the area of the renal tubules from which they originate but typically are small and cuboidal in appearance.

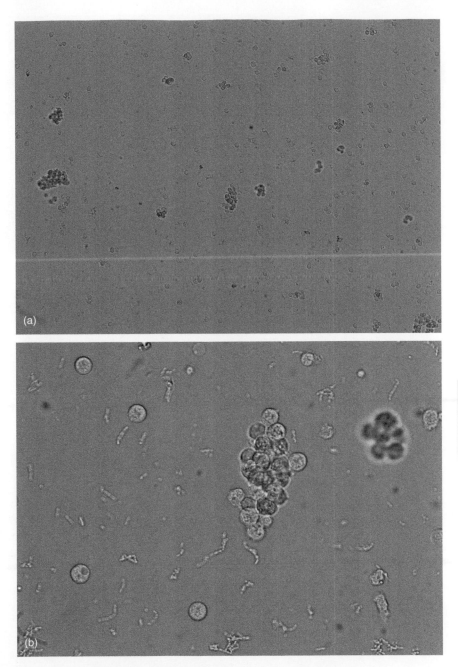

Figure 5.6 WBC clumps with bacteria, (a) 10×; (b) 40×.

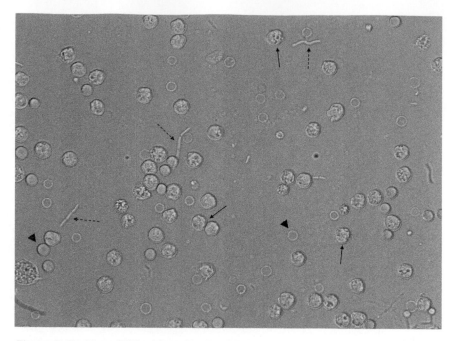

Figure 5.7 Many RBCs (arrowheads), WBCs (arrows), and bacteria (dashed arrows), 40×.

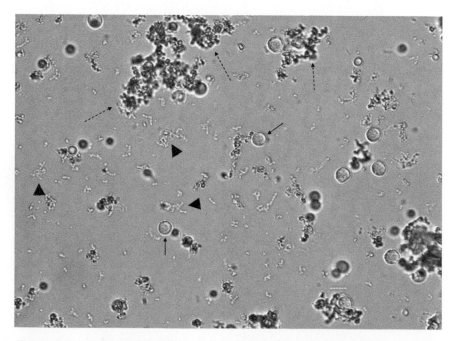

Figure 5.8 Aged sample with bacterial overgrowth. Scattered RBCs (arrows), aggregates of amorphous crystals (dashed arrows), many bacteria (arrowheads), few lipid droplets, 40×.

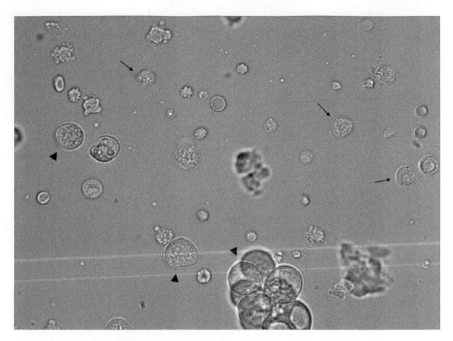

Figure 5.9   WBCs (arrows) with transitional epithelial cells (arrowheads), 40×. (Courtesy of Donna Burton)

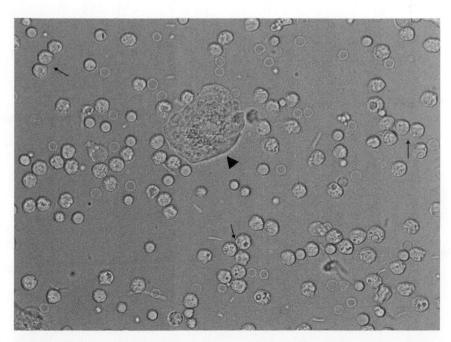

Figure 5.10   Many RBCs, WBCs (arrows), and bacterial rods, one squamous epithelial cell (arrowhead).

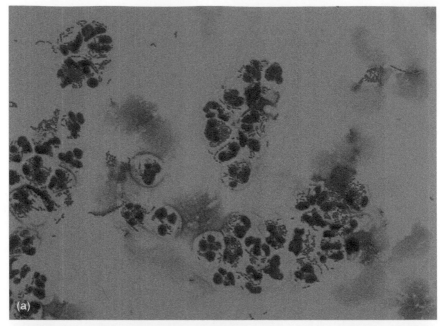

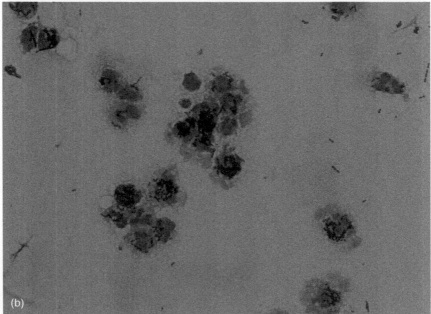

Figure 5.11 (a) Urinary tract infection, many WBCs, and intra- and extracellular bacterial rods. Air-dried and stained urine sediment, Diff-Quik, 50×; (b) urinary tract infection, bacterial rods stain gram positive (dark purple), air-dried and stained urine sediment, Gram stain, 50×.

Squamous epithelial cells

Squamous epithelial cells (SECs) originate from the lining of the urogenital tract, either the urethra or vagina, and are present in free-catch urine samples as a result of tissue sloughing from normal cell turnover and/or in samples collected via urinary tract catheterization. Their presence has no pathological significance unless they are found in large numbers. SECs are the largest cells found in normal urine sediment and appear as large flat cells with a single nucleus and abundant cytoplasm. SECs can be present individually and in variably sized sheets. Occasionally, cells begin to disintegrate or fold and may resemble a large a cast, but routinely, SECs are easy to identify (Figure 5.12a–d).

Transitional epithelial (urothelial) cells

Transitional epithelial cells (TECs) are smaller than SECs but larger than RTEs and are less frequently identified in urine sediment than SECs. These cells arise from portions of the urethra, bladder, ureters, and renal pelves; some glands in the prostate are also lined by TECs. Morphologic variety is caused by the ability of the cell to absorb water and stretching of cells by a full bladder. Various forms of TECs include round, oval, and, less often, caudate to polyhedral. Increased numbers of transitional cells may be present within urine sediment secondary to hyperplastic transitional epithelium of the bladder. Hyperplasia can result from inflammation with or without infection as well as polyps. Cells will be cuboidal, round or ovoid, and fairly uniform in appearance. Columnar-shaped caudate TECs are thought to arise from more proximal portions of the urinary tract rather than the bladder and urethra. The significance of increased numbers of these cells is not entirely clear but may suggest disease within the kidney or ureter (Figure 5.13a–d). Transitional cell carcinoma is a result of neoplastic transformation of TECs and can arise from any place in the urinary tract these cells are present. Urine sediment will reveal numerous variably sized clusters of highly pleomorphic TECs. Urine cytology of an air-dried stained specimen is often necessary for definitive diagnosis. Cytologic features that would support neoplasia in a stained specimen include marked variability in cell and nuclear size, bi- and multi-nucleation with variably sized nuclei within the same cell, prominent, multiple, variably sized, and/or angular nucleoli within a single nucleus, and mitotic figures (Figure 5.14a–c).

Casts

The presence of casts within urine sediment is termed cylindruria (Stockham and Scott 2008). Casts are cylindrical with parallel sides and are the same diameter throughout the length of the cast. They are aptly named as they reflect a cast of the renal tubular lumen. Casts are most likely to form in the distal nephron, either in the distal and collecting tubules, given the higher

Chapter 5

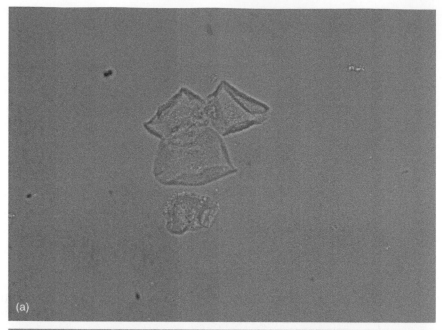

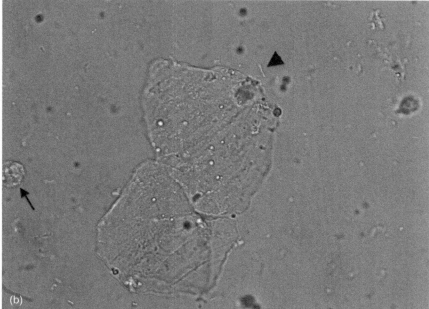

Figure 5.12 (a) Squamous epithelial cells, 40× (Courtesy of Donna Burton); (b) squamous epithelial cells amid a background of many bacteria (arrowhead), WBC (arrow), free-catch urine sample, 40×; (c) squamous epithelial cells and bacteria. Same case as 5.12b, 40×; (d) squamous epithelial cells, urine obtained via catherization, air-dried and stained urine sediment, Wright Giemsa, 20×.

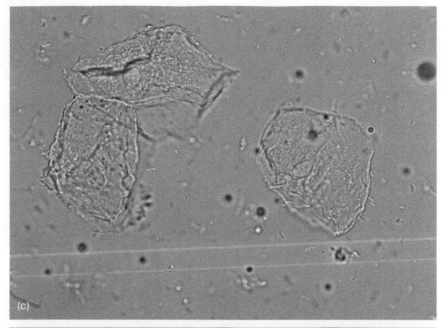

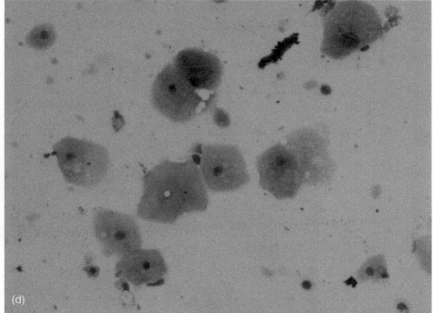

Figure 5.12 (*Continued*)

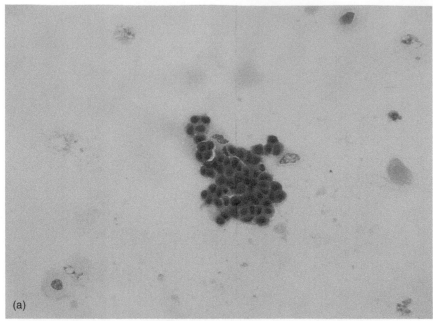

(a)

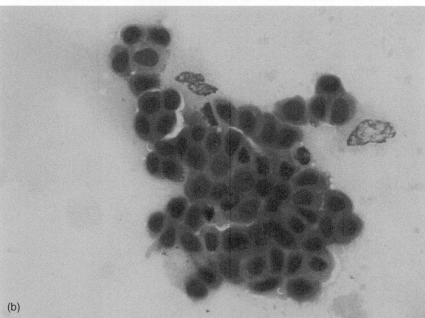

(b)

Figure 5.13 (a) Transitional epithelial cells. Increased numbers of uniform-appearing transitional epithelial cells may result from inflammation, infection, or polyps, air-dried and stained urine sediment, Wright Giemsa, 20× (Courtesy of Dr. Reema Patel); (b) transitional epithelial cells. Higher magnification view of 5.13a, air-dried and stained urine sediment, Wright Giesma, 50× (Courtesy of Dr. Reema Patel); (c) columnar-shaped caudate transitional epithelial cells, in the urine from a dog with uncontrolled hypertension and proteinuria, 40×; (d) columnar epithelial cells, same case as 5.13a, air-dried and stained urine sediment, Wright Giemsa, 50×.

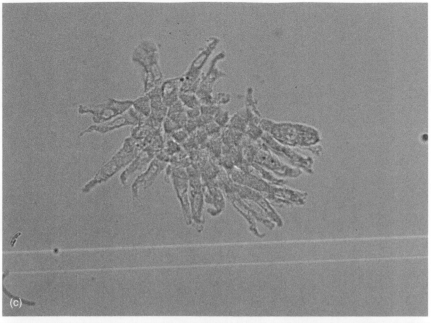

(c)

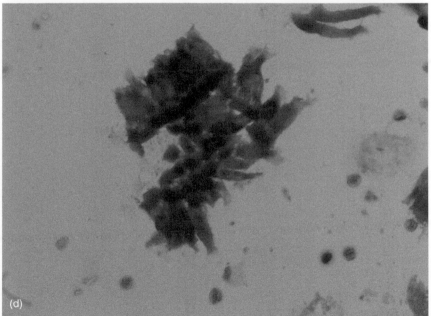

(d)

Figure 5.13 *(Continued)*

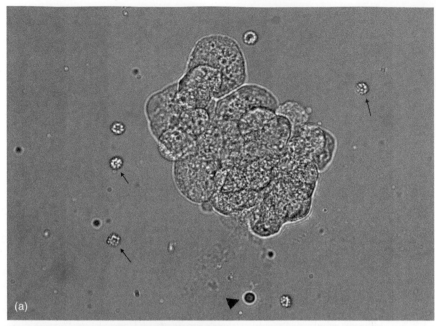

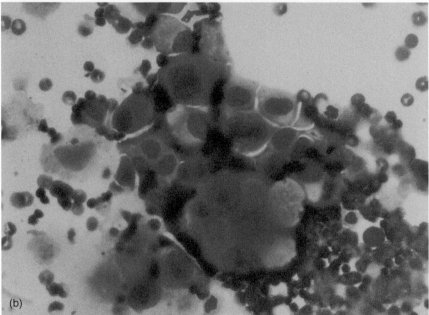

Figure 5.14 (a) Large cluster of neoplastic transitional cells, crenated RBCs (arrows), and lipid droplets (arrowheads), 40×; (b) transitional cell carcinoma, air-dried and stained urine sediment, Diff-Quick, 40×; (c) transitional cell carcinoma, air-dried and stained urine sediment, Wright Giemsa, 40×.

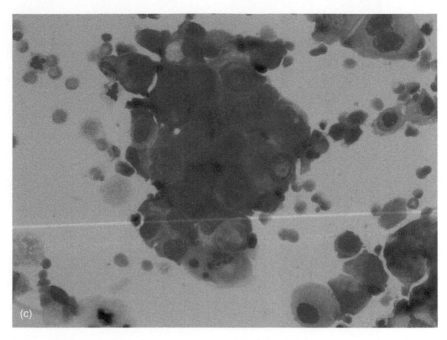

Figure 5.14 *(Continued)*

Chapter 5

urine concentration, but can form in other aspects depending on the underlying etiology. Casts formed in the ascending loop of Henle and the distal convoluted tubule produce structures with tapered ends. The width of the cast is related to the size of the tubule from which it is formed (Stockham and Scott 2008). Structurally proteinaceous and molded from the interior structures of the tubular lumen, any element(s) present in the tubular filtrate can embed or attach to the cast mucoprotein matrix. Casts are classified according to these inclusions, which can be any element. Four conditions contribute to cast formation: increased salt concentration, acidic environment, presence of protein matrix, and tubular fluid stasis (Figures 5.15a–c and 5.16).

RBC Cast

As glomeruli become damaged or diseased or if hemorrhage occurs within the kidney, RBCs and protein can leak into the filtrate. Free RBCs in the urine indicates active bleeding within the urogenital tract (after urine enters the renal pelvis and beyond) while the presence of RBC casts suggest bleeding within the nephron. RBC casts are recognized by their characteristic red-orange color, which originates from the cellular hemoglobin content. As RBC casts age, cells deteriorate but the red-orange hue remains. Large numbers of RBCs in the urine sediment must be examined closely for the presence of

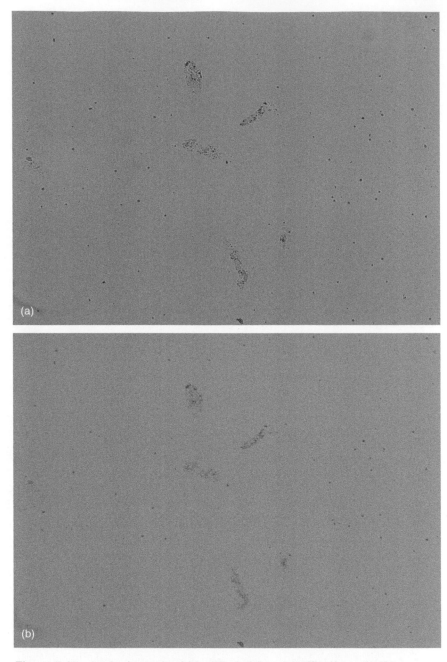

Figure 5.15 (a) Casts are best identified at low magnification with the condenser lowered, 10×; (b) casts are more faint due to an incorrectly raised condenser, 10×; (c) casts (same image as 5.15a), as well as background lipid, are easier to identify when the condenser is lowered, providing more contrast to the specimen, 10×.

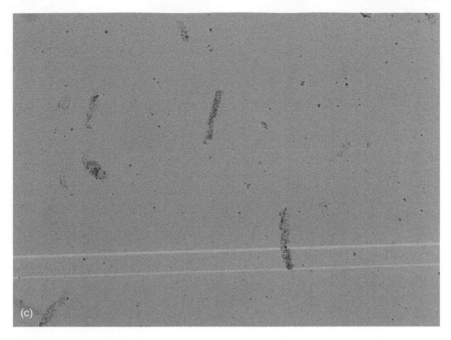

(c)

Figure 5.15 *(Continued)*

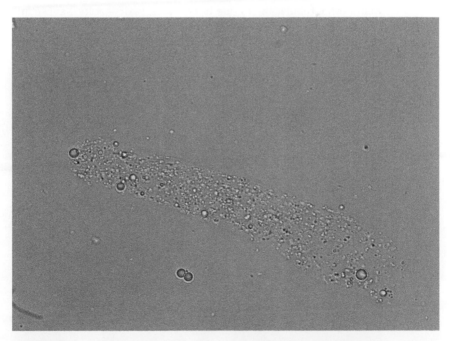

Figure 5.16 High magnification (40×) of unstained urine sediment is used for identification of casts by evaluating cast contents. Although there is lipid within this cast, the mucoprotein matrix suggests it is a hyaline cast, 40×.

mucoprotein matrix to support identification of RBC casts; RBC clumps can be easily mistaken for RBC casts.

WBC Cast

WBC or leukocyte casts result from inflammation involving the renal tubules. They are most frequently composed of neutrophils, so their appearance is granular with multilobed nuclei attached to the mucoprotein matrix. Supravital staining enhances nuclear detail and can assist in identification. Irregular borders occur with increased numbers of WBCs; staining may be necessary to demonstrate characteristic nuclei and is particularly helpful for differentiating WBC casts from RTE casts. As increased numbers of WBCs often clump and can be mistaken for WBC casts, so it is imperative that the mucoprotein cast matrix is visualized.

Epithelial cell cast

Epithelial cell casts, also commonly referred to as cellular casts, result from degeneration of renal tubular epithelial cells. Disintegration of these casts into coarsely and finely granular material is purely a function of time and infers stasis within the nephron. The presence of epithelial cell casts suggests acute renal tubular injury due to necrosis, toxic insults, severe inflammation, hypoperfusion, or hypoxemia (Figure 5.17).

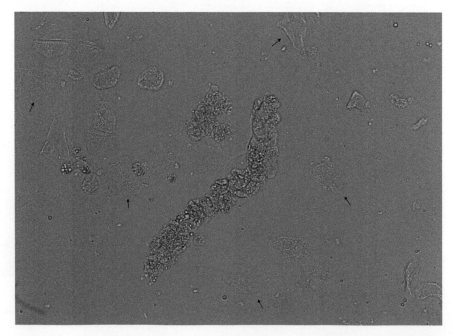

Figure 5.17 Cellular cast amid numerous squamous epithelial cells (arrows), 20×.

Granular cast

Granular casts exhibit a variety of textural consistency. Both coarsely and finely granular casts are frequently seen in urinary sediment. While it is not always necessary to distinguish between coarsely and finely granular casts, many laboratories report this differentiation (Figures 5.18 and 5.19). Once again, it is important to visualize the mucoprotein cast matrix, as amorphous clumps or fecal debris can be mistaken for granular casts. The presence of granular casts, similar to epithelial cell casts, supports underlying, and potentially severe, renal tubular injury. Low numbers, <2/lpf, of granular casts are occasionally seen in urine sediment from healthy animals or slightly increased numbers following exercise (Stockham and Scott 2008). In cases of acute anuric renal failure, urinary stasis may prohibit excretion of casts and cellular material so the absence of granular or cellular casts does not rule out renal tubular injury.

Waxy cast

As granular casts remain in the tubules for extended periods, granule disintegration intensifies, and the cast matrix develops a waxy appearance. Waxy casts are gray, yellow, or colorless. They are highly refractile, broad in width and appear very jagged, broken, or brittle in consistency, displaying irregular clefts. The diameter becomes broader, and ends occasionally have a cork

Chapter 5

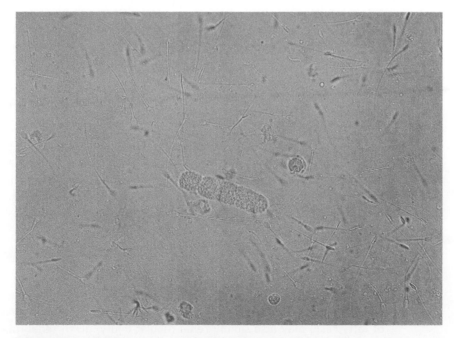

Figure 5.18 Finely granular cast with many spermatozoa, 40×.

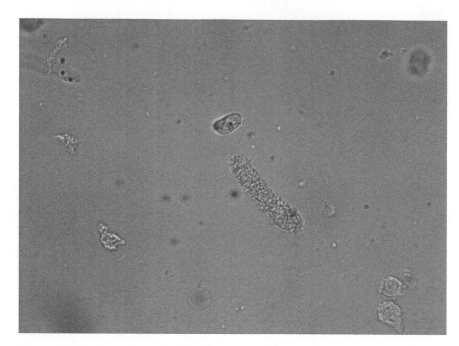

Figure 5.19 Granular cast, 20×. (Courtesy of Donna Burton)

screw appearance. These casts result from extreme urine stasis; the waxy cast matrix is surmised to result from degeneration of cellular or granular hyaline casts. Supravital cytodiagnostic stains tinge waxy casts pink. Waxy casts are attributed to prior renal tubular damage with resulting tubular stasis (Figure 5.20).

Broad cast

Broad casts are up to six times wider than hyaline casts and can be of any cast type, although waxy and granular predominate. Molded from the distal convoluted tubules, broad casts indicate the destruction or widening of the tubule walls. These casts are believed to appear in the collecting tubules as a result of extreme urinary stasis, presumably due to severe renal disease (Chew and DiBartola 2004) (Figure 5.21).

Fatty cast

These casts contain fat droplets or oval fat bodies within the mucoprotein matrix. They are highly refractile using bright field microscopy. The presence of fatty casts may also signify renal tubular injury, given renal tubular epithelial cells contain lipid (Figure 5.22).

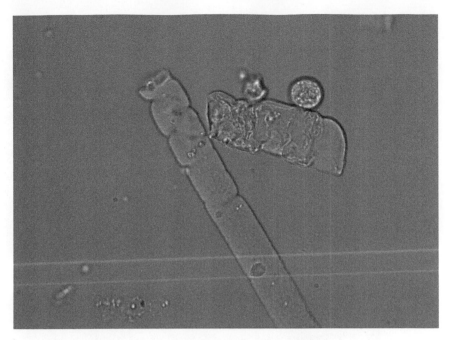

Figure 5.20 Waxy cast, 40×. (Courtesy of Donna Burton)

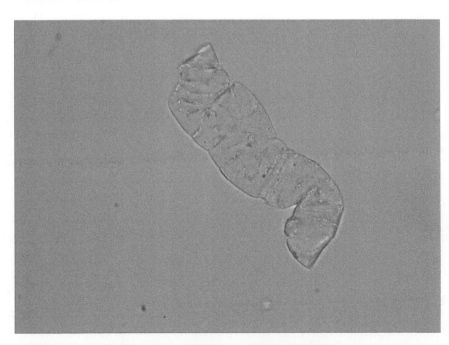

Figure 5.21 Broad cast, 40×. (Courtesy of Donna Burton)

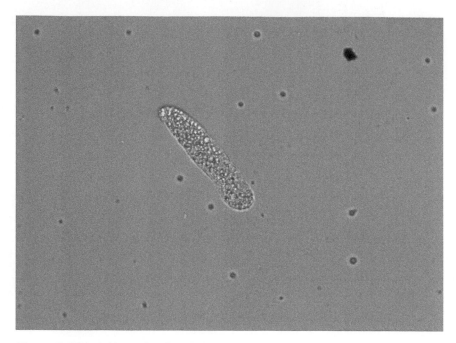

Figure 5.22   Fatty cast, 40×. (Courtesy of Donna Burton)

Hyaline cast

Hyaline casts are colorless, semitransparent casts with typically rounded ends. Best visualized with subdued light, these casts contain no cells, although an occasional adhering cell or granule may be observed but does not alter the classification. Hyaline casts are the most frequently seen cast and are comprised primarily of Tamm–Horsfall protein (uromodulin) normally secreted by distal renal tubular epithelial cells in dogs (Forterre et al. 2004; Stockham and Scott 2008). Rare hyaline casts containing one or two granules are not considered abnormal (Strasinger and DiLorenzo 2008). An occasional recognizable cell is not uncommon. The presence of pathological proteinuria can increase numbers of hyaline casts present in urine sediment (Figures 5.23 and 5.24).

Bacterial cast

Identification of bacterial casts can be challenging, as casts filled with bacteria can resemble granular casts. Gram stain or Diff-Quik staining of the sediment verifies the presence of bacteria-laden casts. Bacterial casts are an infrequent finding; the presence of bacterial casts suggests severe renal tubular infection.

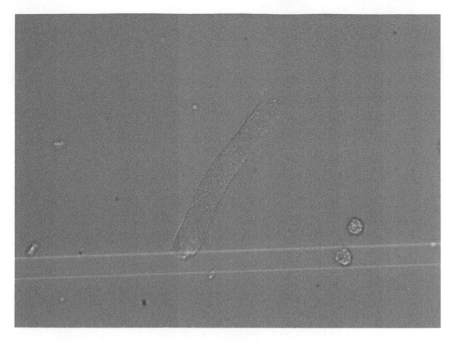

Figure 5.23 Hyaline cast, 40×. (Courtesy of Donna Burton)

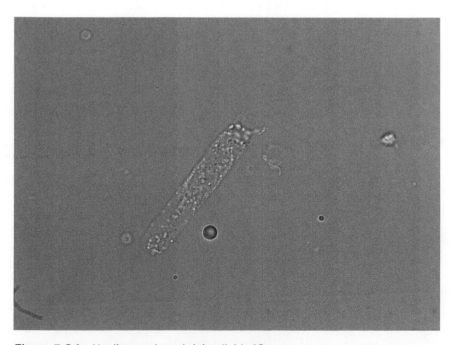

Figure 5.24 Hyaline cast containing lipid, 40×.

Mixed cellular casts

Casts can contain a mixture of any cells present in the urinary filtrate, and casts containing multiple cell combinations are possible.

Crystals

A variety of crystals can be found in urine sediment, most with unique appearance and solubility characteristics. The presence of many crystals is non-pathological, although some crystals possess clinical significance, necessitating microscopic identification.

Crystal formation

Crystals are formed by precipitation of solutes, specifically inorganic salts, organic compounds, or iatrogenic compounds (Strasinger and DiLorenzo 2008). Crystals are more likely to form in concentrated urine samples. Decreased temperature enhances the precipitation of crystals, so refrigerated specimens often incur this *in vitro* interference. Unfortunately, formed crystals obscure other clinically significant microscopic elements. This pre-analytic nuisance can be reversed by allowing the urine specimen to warm to room temperature prior to analysis. Crystal formation is also affected by urine concentration, and crystalluria in freshly voided urine specimens is associated with concentrated specimens.

Crystal identification

The most frequently encountered crystals possess characteristic shapes and colors, although the pH of urine specimens may assist in identification of urine crystals because this influences the type of chemicals precipitated (Strasinger and DiLorenzo 2008). An acidic environment favors crystallization of organic and iatrogenic compounds, while inorganic salts are less soluble in neutral and alkaline environments (with the exception of calcium oxalate which precipitates in both acidic and neutral urine). Chemically counteracting these properties in the laboratory causes crystals to dissolve, and these solubility characteristics can assist in crystal identification. Astute microscopists aliquot sediment specimens for chemical evaluation as necessary. Descriptions of frequently visualized crystals and their solubility properties can be found in Table 5.5. Clinical significance of many of these crystals can be found in Table 5.6. (Figures 5.25–5.39).

The Lignin test confirms the presence of sulfonamide-induced crystalluria. In the presence of sulfa drug metabolites, a drop of urine sediment on newspaper with one to two drops of dilute HCl added produces a bright yellow orange color (Gregory 2003).

Table 5.5 Characteristics of crystals found in urine sediment

Name	Appearance	Urine pH favoring formation	Solubility characteristics	
			Soluble in:	Insoluble in:
Ammonium (bi) urate	Brown, three-dimensional spheres with either smooth edges or irregular, horn-like projections ("thorny apple"); individual or clusters	Alkaline, neutral, or slightly acidic	Acetic acid 10% NaOH Strong alkali	
Amorphous phosphate (magnesium, calcium)	Colorless to yellow-brown, fine granules With centrifugation, pellet is white.	Alkaline	Acetic acid	Alkaline
Amorphous urate (calcium, magnesium, sodium, potassium)	Colorless to yellow-brown, fine granules With centrifugation, pellet is pink-tinged.	Acidic	Alkaline	Acetic acid
Bilirubin	Amber, branching needles resembling twigs or antlers	Acidic	Acid Alkali Acetone	Alcohol
Calcium carbonate	Colorless to yellow, spherical or dumbbell shapes Rule out for dumbbell shape: Ca oxalate monohydrate	Alkaline or neutral	Acetic acid (effervesces when added)	
Calcium oxalate: dihydrate	Colorless, refractile, three-dimensional octahedron, mail-type envelope	Acidic, but any pH possible	Dilute HCl	Acetic acid
Calcium oxalate: monohydrate	Colorless, two-dimensional. Variable forms: six-sided with a "picket fence" or "stake" appearance, dumbbell or ovoid, some flat, elongate; rare: "orzo" or "hemp seed" shape	Acidic, but any pH possible	Dilute HCl	Acetic acid

(Continued)

Table 5.5 *(Continued)*

Name	Appearance	Urine pH favoring formation	Solubility characteristics	
			Soluble in:	Insoluble in:
Calcium phosphate	Formed from: amorphous phosphates and calcium phosphates Colorless, elongate, thin prisms, spheric (dog), +/– pointed end Aggregates or needle-like	Alkaline		
Cholesterol	Colorless, transparent; large, flat rectangular plates with one or more square notched corners	Any	Acetone	
Cystine	Colorless hexagonal plates, can be individual or present in clumps	Acidic	Dilute HCl Ammonia	Acetic acid Acetone Alcohol Heat
Drug-associated (antibiotics)				
Ampicillin	Rare, colorless long prisms that form sheaves (refrigeration accentuates sheave formation)	Acidic	Acetone	
Ciprofloxacin	Yellow to brown, long needle-like crystals forming sheaves, fans, or butterflies	Unknown		Acetic acid 10% NaOH
Sulfonamide	Pale yellow to yellow-brown, aggregates with variable crystal morphology: needles, sheaves, or spherical with radiating spokes (confirm with lignin test)	Acidic	Acetone	
Drug-associated (radiographic contrast agents)	Resemble cholesterol plates or long pointed crystals	Acidic	10% NaOH	

Table 5.5 *(Continued)*

Name	Appearance	Urine pH favoring formation	Solubility characteristics	
			Soluble in:	Insoluble in:
Leucine	Clear to yellow brown spheres with concentric circles and radial striations	Acidic to neutral	10% NaOH	Dilute HCl
Melamine	Brown to green brown circular crystals with radiating striations originating in the center of the crystal			
Triple phosphate (Magnesium ammonium phosphate; Struvite)	Colorless, "coffin-lids"—three to six sided prisms with oblique ends	Any, more so neutral to alkaline	Acetic acid	
Tyrosine	Rare, colorless or yellow fine needles in sheaves or rosettes	Acidic	Ammonium hydroxide Dilute HCl	Acetic acid Alcohol
Uric acid	Rhomboid, oval with pointed ends, prisms; less often 6-sided (hexagonal plate) which gives cystine appearance Note: Acetic acid added to urine with amorphous urates or ammonium (bi)urate crystals may result in uric acid crystal formation.	Acidic	10% NaOH Alkaline	Acetic acid Dilute HCl Heat Alcohol
Xanthine	Similar to ammonium urate or amorphous urates, frequently appear amorphous. Yellow brown to brown, varying-sized spherules.	Not specified		

Sodium hydroxide = NaOH

Hydrochloric acid = HCl

Sources: Data from Albasan et al. (2005); Bannasch et al. (2008); Ben-Ezra et al. (2007); Brandt and Blauvelt (2010); Casal et al. (1995); Case et al. (1992); Cianciolo et al. (2008); Karmi et al. (2010); Mundt and Shanahan (2011); Osborne et al. (2008, 2009); Osborne and Stevens (1999); Pallatto et al. (2005); Puschner et al. (2007); Sink and Feldman (2004); Strasinger and DiLorenzo (2008); Thompson et al. (2008); VanZuilen et al. (1997); Yarlagadda and Perazella (2008).

Table 5.6 Clinical significance of crystals found in urine sediment

Name	Clinical significance
Ammonium (bi)urate	Hyperammonemia due to a portosystemic shunt or hepatic failure.
Amorphous phosphate (magnesium, calcium)	No clinical significance. May form cast-like structures leading to misinterpretation.
Amorphous urate (calcium, magnesium, sodium, potassium)	No clinical significance, formed from salts of uric acid. Increased formation with refrigeration. May form cast-like structures leading to misinterpretation
Bilirubin	Indicate some degree bilirubinuria. Can be normal in highly concentrated urine samples from dogs (low renal threshold for bilirubin). Other causes same as for bilirubinuria.
Calcium carbonate	An expected finding in urine sediment from horses but not dogs or cats. These are seen, however, anecdotally in dogs.
Calcium oxalate: dihydrate	Can be a normal finding in dogs and cats, form in urine samples upon standing. Less often seen in ethylene glycol (EG) toxicosis.
Calcium oxalate: monohydrate	Indicate hyperoxaluric disorders or hypercalciuria. Hyperoxaluria due to ethylene glycol (EG) toxicosis or ingestion of oxalate-rich foods (e.g., peanut butter, sweet potatoes, some whole grains). The absence of these crystals does not rule out EG toxicosis.
Calcium phosphate	Similar to triple phosphate (struvite).
Cholesterol	Suggests cell membrane breakdown as cell membranes are comprised of cholesterol. May be seen with some renal diseases and proteinuria although are not a specific finding.
Cystine	Indicates cystinuria, an inherited defect in urinary cystine transport (decreased reabsorption of cystine from renal tubular lumen). Breeds reported: Newfoundland, English Bulldog, Dachshund, Chihuahua, Mastiff, Australian Cattle Dog, Bullmastiff, American Staffordshire Terrier, and mixed breeds. Less soluble in acidic urine which increases likelihood of urolith formation and obstruction.

Table 5.6 (*Continued*)

Name	Clinical significance

Drug-associated (antibiotics)	Reported with ampicillin, sulfa-containing (sulfonamide crystals), ciprofloxacin (one case report)
	Increased precipitation of crystals due to:
	    Urine that is highly concentrated and of low volume
	    High dose of medication leading to high rate of urinary excretion
	    Low drug solubility (may relate to urine pH)
	Can confirm presence of sulfa crystals with lignin test (see text).

Drug-associated (radiographic contrast agents)	Reported with:
	    Hypaque®
	    Diatrizoate meglumine (Renografin)

Hippuric acid	Rare; significance unknown
Leucine	Rare. In humans associated with severe liver disease, aminoaciduria. Significance in dog: unknown, liver disease also.
Melamine	Identified in patients with acute renal failure that ingested melamine- and cyanuric-contaminated pet food.
Triple phosphate (Magnesium ammonium phosphate; Struvite)	Often of no clinical significance. Can see with urinary tract infection (urease-splitting bacteria). More likely to form in alkaline urine, refrigerated specimens.
Tyrosine	Rare. Associated with severe liver disease in dogs, aminoaciduria (humans); can co-occur with leucine crystals in humans. Note: May be mistaken for bilirubin crystals which are more amber in color with less smooth edges.
Uric acid	Inherited defect in purine metabolism which leads to hyperuricosuria. Dalmations: Considered a "normal" finding. Other predisposed breeds: Bulldog and Black Russian Terrier. Increases risk of uric acid uroliths (stones), especially in acidic urine. Liver disease—hepatic failure or portosystemic shunt. (In the absence of liver disease, consider genetic testing for mutation) Can be normal in acidic urine containing amorphous urates allowed to stand at room temperature. Also, uric acid crystals can result following addition of acetic acid added to urine with amorphous urates or ammonium (bi)urate crystals.

(*Continued*)

Table 5.6 *(Continued)*

Name	Clinical significance
Xanthine	High dose therapy with allopurinol (treatment for hyperuricosuria with decreased conversion of xanthine to uric acid). Also reported in a family of Cavalier King Charles spaniels (in absence of allopurinol).

Sources: Data from Albasan et al. (2005); Bannasch et al. (2008); Ben-Ezra et al. (2007); Brandt and Blauvelt (2010); Casal et al. (1995); Case et al. (1992); Cianciolo et al. (2008); Karmi et al. (2010); Mundt and Shanahan (2011); Osborne et al. (2008, 2009); Osborne and Stevens (1999); Pallatto et al. (2005); Puschner et al. (2007); Sink and Feldman (2004); Strasinger and DiLorenzo (2008); Thompson et al. (2008); VanZuilen et al. (1997); Yarlagadda and Perazella (2008).

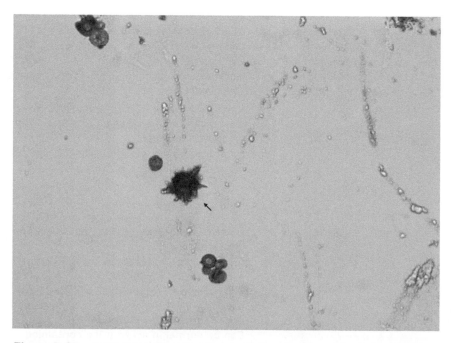

Figure 5.25 Ammonium biurate crystals, both smooth and irregular borders. Arrow points to "thorny apple" form, other smooth forms present individually and in small groups, 20×. (Courtesy of Dr. Reema Patel)

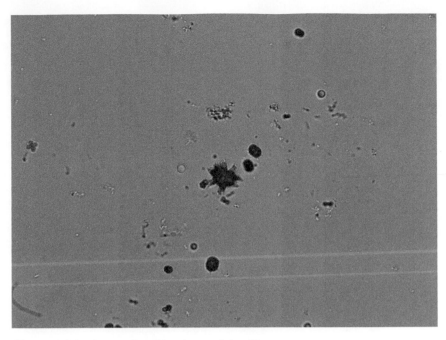

Figure 5.26 Ammonium biurate crystals, 40×.

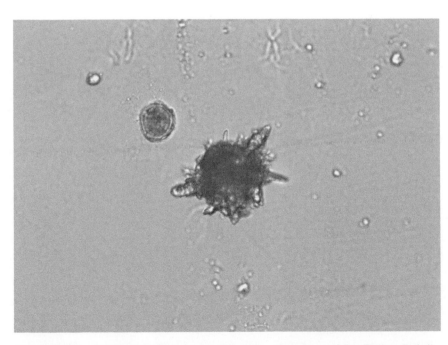

Figure 5.27 Ammonium biurate crystal, 100×. (Courtesy of Dr. Reema Patel)

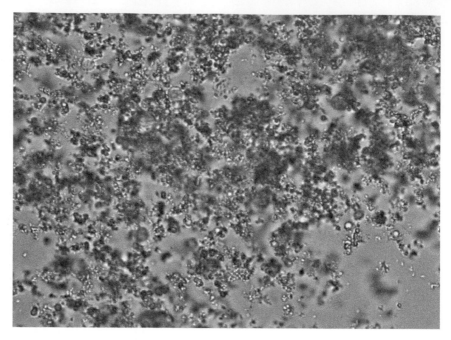

Figure 5.28   Amorphous crystals, 40×.

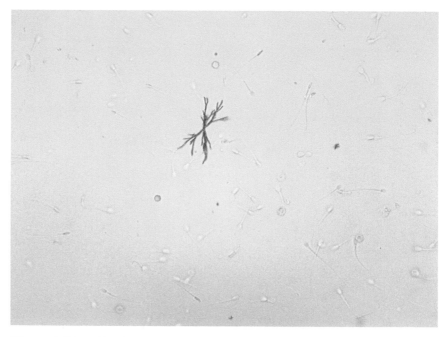

Figure 5.29   Bilirubin crystal with numerous spermatozoa, 40×. (Courtesy of Donna Burton)

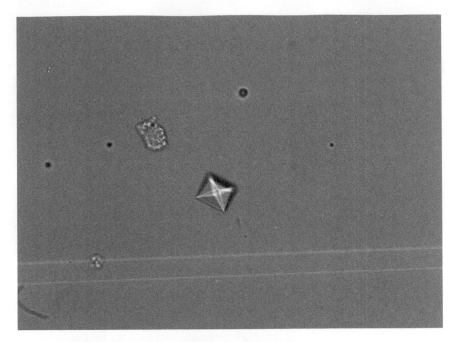

Figure 5.30   Calcium oxalate dihydrate crystal, 40×.

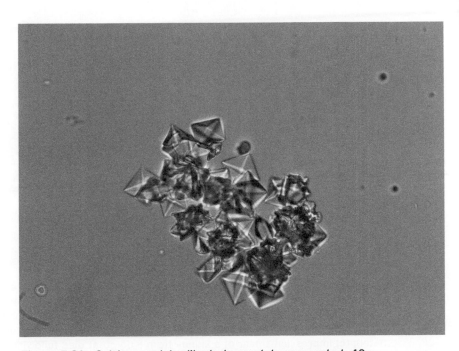

Figure 5.31   Calcium oxalate dihydrate crystals aggregated, 40×.

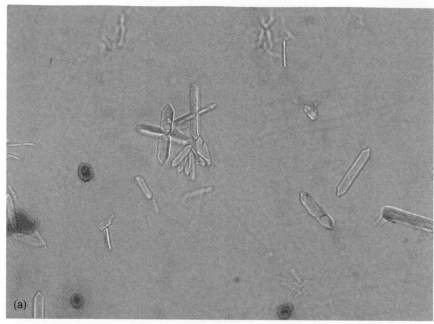

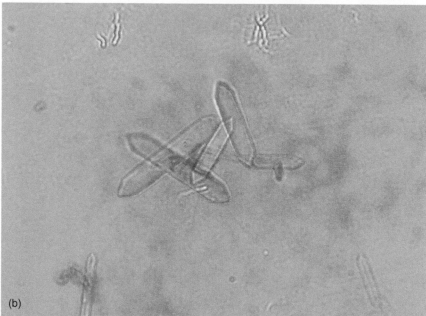

Figure 5.32 (a) Calcium oxalate monohydrate crystals, "picket fence" appearance, in the urine from a patient with ethylene glycol toxicity, Wright Giemsa, 50× (Courtesy of Dr. Reema Patel); (b) calcium oxalate monohydrate crystals, same case as 5.32a, Wright Giemsa, 100× (Courtesy of Dr. Reema Patel); (c) impression smear of a kidney from a dog that died following ethylene glycol intoxication. "Picket fence" crystal (arrow) and "dumbbell" calcium oxalate monohydrate crystal (arrowhead) shapes present amid numerous renal epithelial cells and bare nuclei, Wright Giemsa, 40×; (d) "hemp seed" or "orzo" shape of calcium oxalate monohydrate crystal (arrow), 40×.

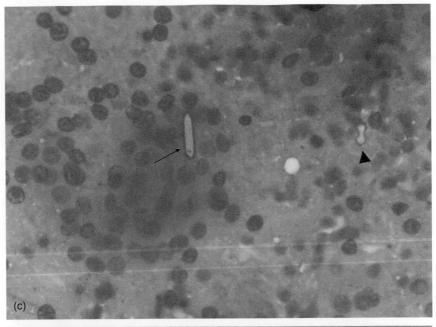

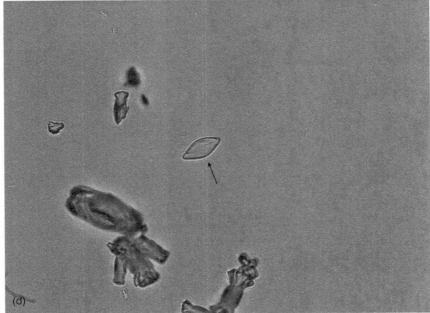

Figure 5.32 (*Continued*)

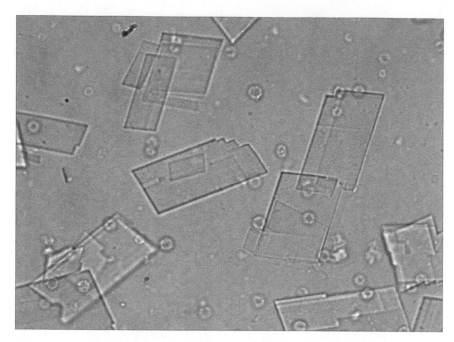

Figure 5.33 Cholesterol crystal, 40×. (Courtesy of Donna Burton)

Bacteria

Both bacilli or cocci can be found in urine sediment, although identification should be confirmed with staining of air-dried sediment smears (Diff-Quick and/or Gram stain) and/or culture. Organisms are usually motile; however, cocci can frequently be mistaken for amorphous crystals. Bacilli are typically easy to identify, especially if mature forms are present (Figure 5.40).

Yeast or fungi

Although morphologically similar to both RBCs and lipid, when viewed microscopically, yeast are ovoid rather than round. Yeast are colorless, refractile, variable in size, and frequently exhibit budding. In severe infections, mycelia (hyphal structures) may be observed. When differentiation from RBCs cannot be visualized, addition of acetic acid to urine sediment will lyse RBCs while leaving yeast intact. *Candida* sp. is more frequently identified as it is considered normal flora of the urogenital tract. Increased numbers can result from underlying urinary tract disease, recent antibiotic treatment, and glucosuria due to diabetes mellitus (Figures 5.41a,b and 5.42). Fungal infections due to blastomycosis, cryptococcosis, coccidioidomycosis, and aspergillosis rarely manifest in urine specimens; if present, they reflect systemic fungal disease

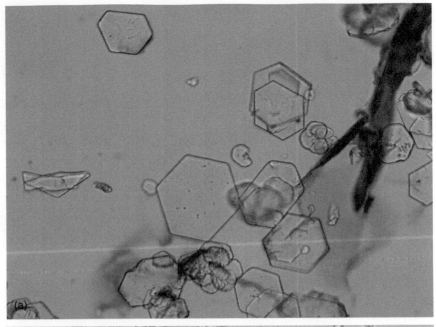

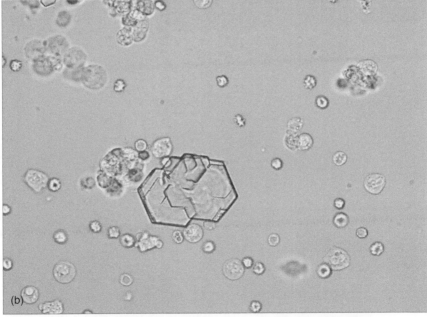

Figure 5.34 (a) Cystine crystal in the urine from a dog with cystinuria, Wright Giemsa, 40×; (b) cystine crystals, aggregated, with RBCs, WBCs, and few larger epithelial cells, 40×.

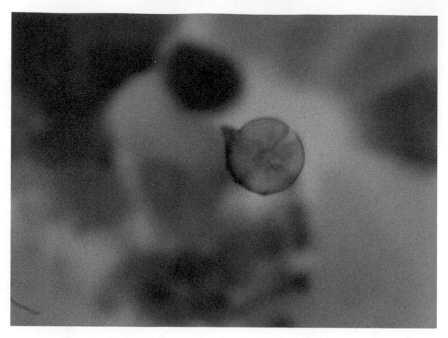

Figure 5.35   Leucine-like crystal from a dog with severe hepatitis, Wright Giemsa, 100×.

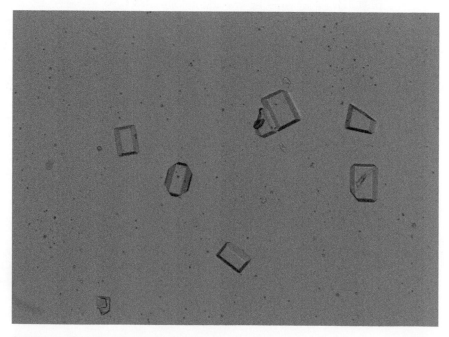

Figure 5.36   Struvite crystal, 10×.

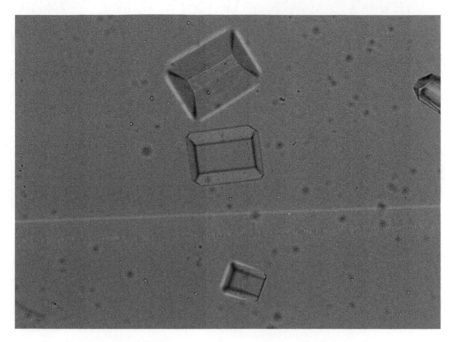

Figure 5.37   Struvite crystal, 20×.

with renal involvement. Only aspergillosis presents in the hyphal form. *Candida* sp. may display formation of pseudohyphae. Stained air-dried sediment specimens may allow for better evaluation of yeast or fungal components.

Parasites

Parasite ova may be seen in urine sediment as a result of fecal contamination and, less often, parasitic infections; they are large elements with distinctive forms. They can be visualized from low magnification and should not be confused with plant pollen (see "Contaminants and Artifacts" section below). Parasites that could be seen in a urine sediment include *Dirofilaria immitis* microfilaria (heartworm disease), *Dioctophyma renale* (giant kidney worm of the dog), and *Pearsonema* (*Capillaria*) sp. (bladder worm of the dog and cat) (Stockham and Scott 2008) (Figures 5.43 and 5.44).

Mucus

Mucus appears as fine thread-like strands possessing low refractive index when viewed using subdued light with bright field microscopy. Frequently

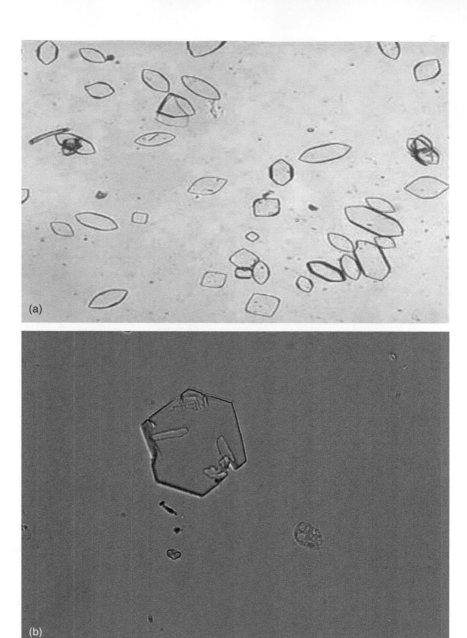

Figure 5.38 (a) Uric acid crystals, 10× (Courtesy of Dr. Patricia McManus); (b) uric acid (cystine-like) crystal from a male bulldog with hyperuricosuria and uroliths, 40×.

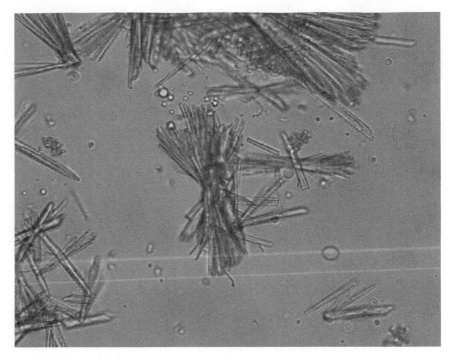

Figure 5.39 Ciprofloxacin crystals, 40×. (Courtesy of Drs. Carolina Escobar and Carol Grindem)

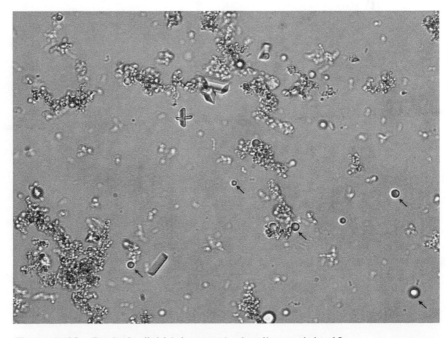

Figure 5.40 Bacteria, lipid (at arrows), struvite crystals, 40×.

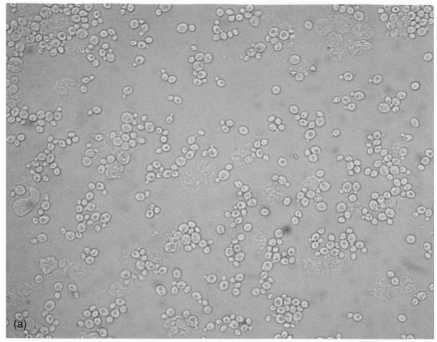

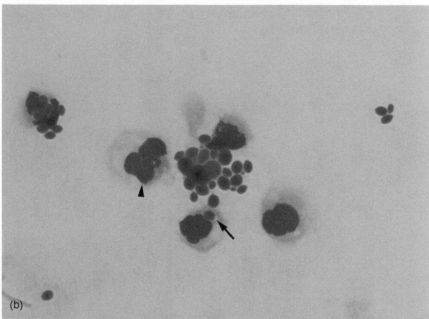

Figure 5.41 (a) Numerous yeast (*Candida* sp.) with frequent budding from a diabetic cat, 60×; (b) many ovoid, darkly basophilic yeast (*Candida* sp.) and poorly preserved neutrophils (arrowhead), some yeast present within neutrophils (arrow), air-dried and stained urine sediment, Wright Giemsa, 100×.

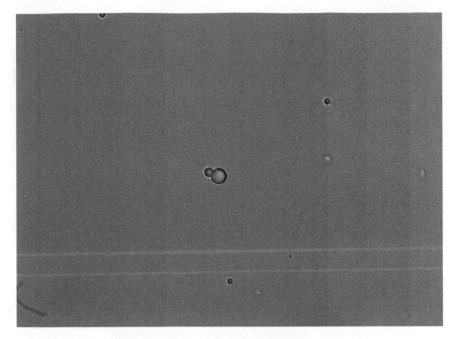

Figure 5.42 Lipid mimicking budding yeast. Note that lipid lacks internal structure, 40×.

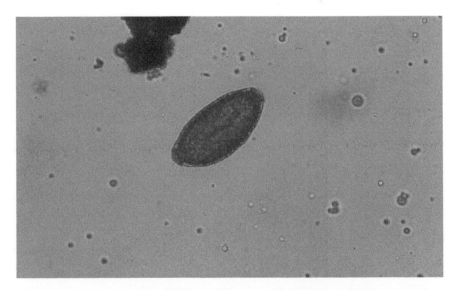

Figure 5.43 *Pearsonema (Capillaria) feliscati* egg (bladder worm) in the urine (stained) from a cat. High magnification reveals the terminal plugs (at either end) which are slightly angled. (Courtesy of Dr. Anne Zajac)

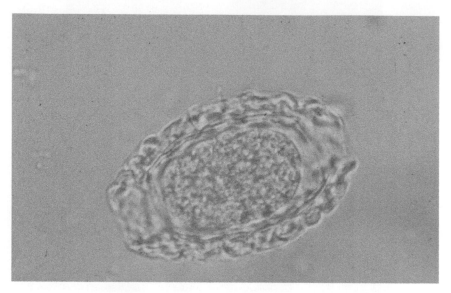

Figure 5.44 *Dioctophyma renale,* high magnification of egg of the giant kidney worm of dogs. (Courtesy of Dr. Anne Zajac)

confused with hyaline casts, mucus threads are longer and irregular in shape. As single threads or en masse, mucus is found in the background of the visual field, with other formed elements taking the forefront. Mucus is proteinaceous and is produced by epithelial cells of the lower genitourinary tract and RTE cells. Tamm-Horsfall protein is a major constituent of mucus.

Spermatozoa

The characteristic traits of spermatozoa are its long flagella-like tail attached to an oval body by a central rectangular mid-piece. Spermatozoa may be motile or stationary but rarely exhibit motility in urine sediment. The presence of spermatozoa is considered an expected finding in the urine collected from intact male dogs.

Contaminants and artifacts

A wide variety of contaminants and artifacts can challenge even experienced microscopists (Figures 5.45 and 5.46). Contaminants may include dust particles, hair, starch granules, glass shards, cotton and wool fibers, and pollen (Figures 5.47–5.54).

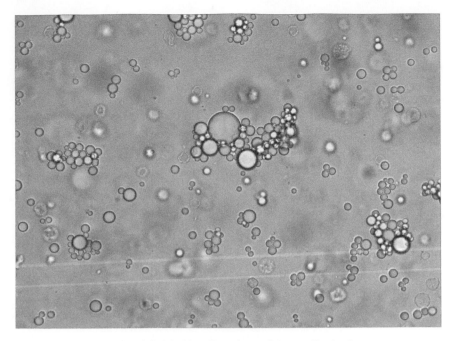

Figure 5.45 Abundant lipid, 40×. (Courtesy of Donna Burton)

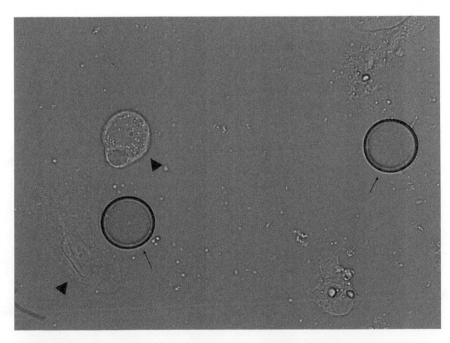

Figure 5.46 Air bubbles (arrows) trapped under the coverslip, squamous epithelial cells (arrowheads), 40×.

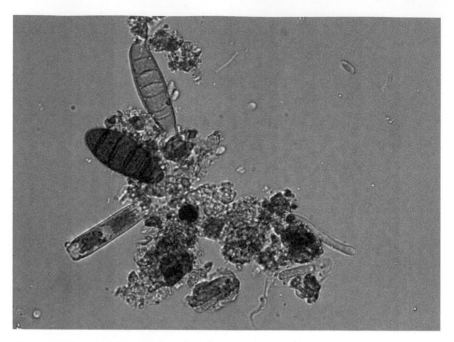

Figure 5.47 Various fungal conidia contaminants amid amorphous debris and few bacteria in a free-catch urine sample from a dog, 40×.

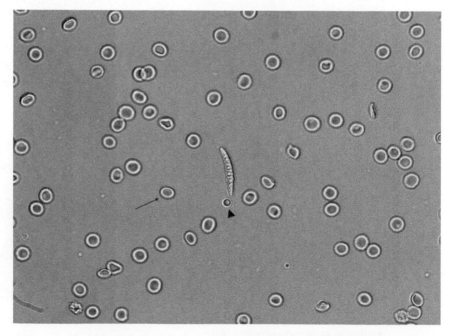

Figure 5.48 An elongate fungal conidia (center), many RBCs (arrow), and free lipid (arrowhead), 40×.

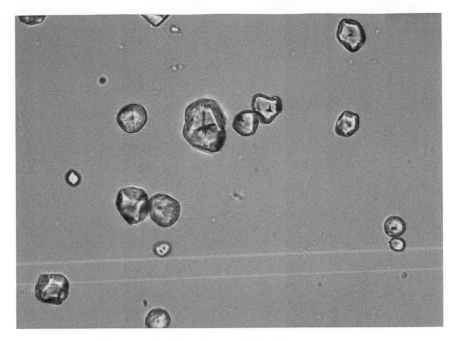

Figure 5.49 Glove powder (starch granules), 40×.

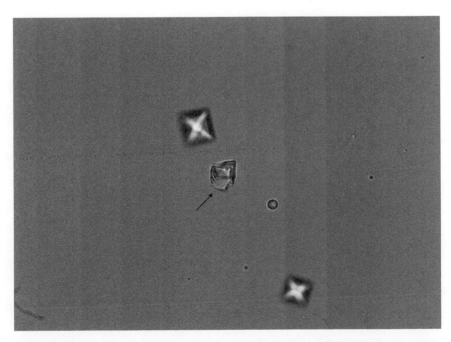

Figure 5.50 Glass shards (arrow) between two calcium oxalate dihydate and lipid droplet, 40×.

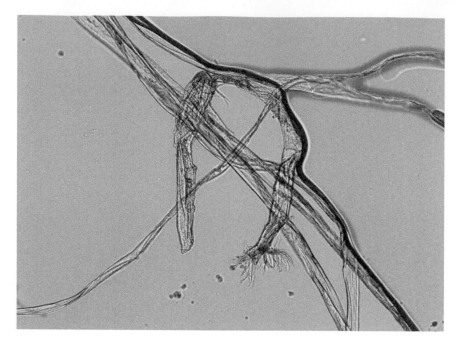

Figure 5.51   Cotton fibers, 20×.

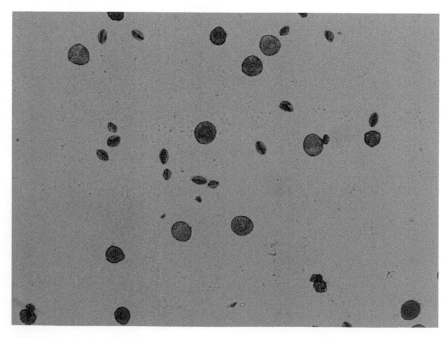

Figure 5.52   Pollen, 10×.

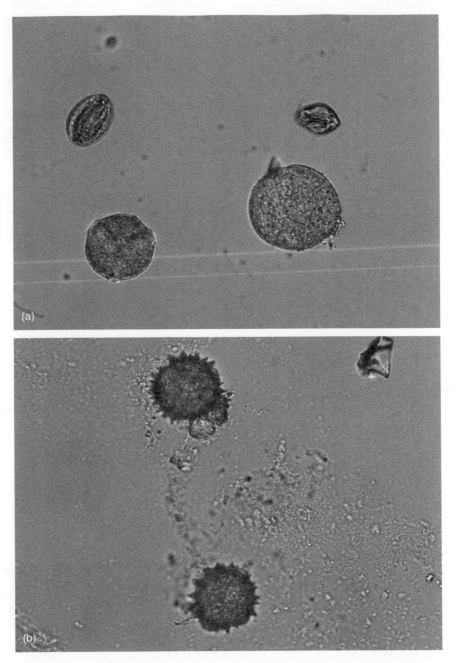

Figure 5.53 (a–d) Pollen 40×.

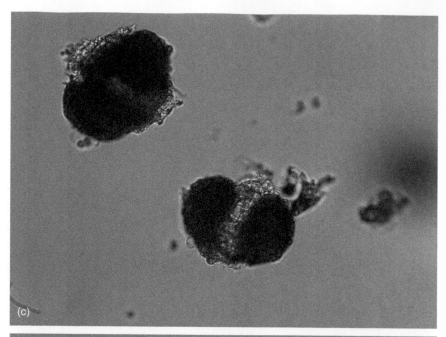

(c)

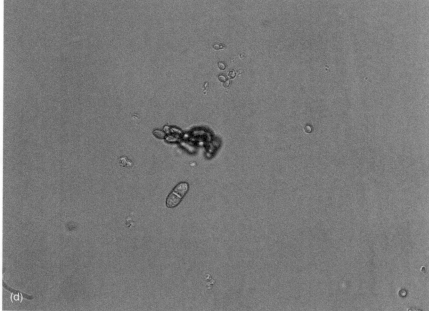

(d)

Figure 5.53 (*Continued*) (c) Pine pollen, 40×; (d) fine pollen particulate debris, 40×.

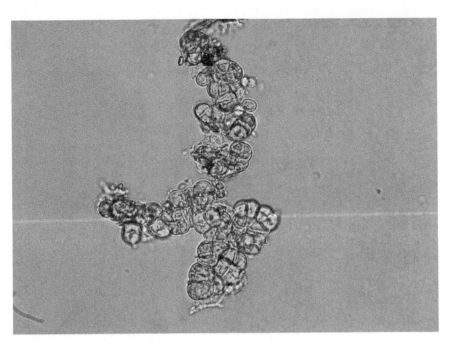

Figure 5.54 Plant material, likely chloroplasts, 40×.

References

Albasan H, Lulich JP, Osborne CA, Lekcharoensuk C. 2005. Evaluation of the association between sex and risk of forming urate uroliths in Dalmatians. *Journal of the Veterinary Medical Association* **227**(4): 565-9.

Bannasch D, Safra N, Young A, Karmi N, Schaible RS, Ling GV. 2008. Mutations in the SLC2A9 gene cause hyperuricosuria and hyperuricemia in the dog. *PLoS Genetics* **4**(11): e1000246. doi:10.1371/journal.pgen.1000246.

Ben-Ezra J, Zhao S, McPherson R. 2007. Basic examination of urine. In *Henry's Clinical Diagnosis and Management by Laboratory Methods*, 21st ed. McPherson RA, Pincus MR, eds., pp. 393-409. Philadelphia: Saunders Elsevier.

Brandt LE, Blauvelt MM. 2010. What is your diagnosis? Urine sediment from a Southern California cat with weight loss. *Veterinary Clinical Pathology* **39**(4): 517-8.

Casal ML, Giger U, Bovee KC, Patterson DF. 1995. Inheritance of cystinuria and renal defect in Newfoundland. *Journal of the American Veterinary Association* **207**(12): 1585-9.

Case LC, Ling GV, Franti CE, Ruby AL, Stevens F, Johnson DL. 1992. Cystine-containing urinary calculi in dogs: 102 cases (1981-1989). *Journal of the American Veterinary Association* **201**(1): 129-33.

Chew DJ, DiBartola SP. 2004. Urinalysis interpretation. In *Interpretation of Canine and Feline Urinalysis*. Chew DJ, DiBartola SP, eds., p. 29. Wilmington, NC: The Gloyd Group.

Cianciolo RE, Bischoff K, Ebel JG, Van Winkle TJ, Goldstein RE, Serfilippi LM. 2008. Clinicopathologic, histologic, and toxicologic findings in 70 cats inadvertently exposed to pet food contaminated with melamine and cyanuric acid. *Journal of the American Veterinary Association* **233**(5): 729-37.

Chapter 5

Forterre S, Raila J, Schweigert FJ. 2004. Protein profiling of urine from dogs with renal disease using ProteinChip analysis. *Journal of Veterinary Diagnostic Investigation* **16**(4): 271-7.

Free HM. 1986. *Modern Urine Chemistry*. 5th printing. Ames, IA: Miles Laboratories, Inc.

Gregory CR. 2003. Urinary system. In *Duncan & Prasse's Veterinary Laboratory Medicine Clinical Pathology*, 4th ed. Latimer KS, Mahaffe EA, Prasse KW, eds., pp. 231-59. Ames, IA: Iowa State Press.

Karmi N, Brown EA, Hughes SS, McLaughlin B, Mellersh CS, Biourge V, Bannasch DL. 2010. Estimated frequency of the canine hyperuricosuria mutation in different dog breeds. *Journal of Veterinary Internal Medicine* **24**(6): 1337-42.

Mundt L, Shanahan K. 2011. Microscopic examination of urinary sediment. In *Graff's Textbook of Routine Urinalysis and Body Fluids*, 2nd ed. Mundt L, Shanahan K, eds., pp. 62-8. Philadelphia: Lippincott Williams and Wilkins.

Osborne CA, Stevens J. 1999. Urine sediment: under the microscope. In *Urinalysis: A Clinical Guide to Compassionate Patient Care*. Osborne CA, Stevens J, eds., pp. 125-50. Shawnee, KS: Bayer Corporation.

Osborne CA, Lulich JP, Swanson LL, Swanson LL, Albasan H. 2008. Drug-induced urolithiasis. *Veterinary Clinics North America. Small Animal Practice* **39**(1): 55-63.

Osborne CA, Lulich JP, Ulrich LK, Koehler LA, Albasan H, Sauer L, Schubert G. 2009. Melamine and cyanuric acid-induced crystalluria, uroliths, and nephrotoxicity in dogs and cats. *Veterinary Clinics North America. Small Animal Practice* **39**(1): 1-14.

Pallatto V, Wood M, Grindem C. 2005. Urine sediment from a Chihuahua. *Veterinary Clinical Pathology* **34**(4): 425-8.

Puschner B, Poppenga RH, Lowenstine LJ, Filigenzi MS, Pesavento PA. 2007. Assessment of melamine and cyanuric acid toxicity in cats. *Journal of Veterinary Diagnostic Investigation* **19**(6): 616-24.

Sink CA, Feldman BF. 2004. Microscopic analysis. In *Laboratory Urinalysis and Hematology for the Small Animal Practitioner*. Sink CA, Feldman BF, eds., pp. 20-44. Jackson, WY: Teton NewMedia.

Stockham SL, Scott MA. 2008. Urinary system. In *Fundamentals of Veterinary Clinical Pathology*, 2nd ed. Stockham SL, Scott MA, eds., pp. 426-33. Ames, IA: Blackwell Publishing.

Strasinger SK, DiLorenzo MS. 2008. Microscopic examination of urine. In *Urinalysis and Body Fluids*, 5th ed. Strasinger SK, DiLorenzo M, eds. pp. 81-126. Philadelphia: FA Davis Company.

Thompson ME, Lewin-Smith MR, Kalasinsky VF, Pizzolato KM, Fleetwood ML, McElhaney MR, Johnson TO. 2008. Characterization of melamine-containing and calcium oxalate crystals in three dogs with suspected pet food-induced nephrotoxicosis. *Veterinary Pathology* **45**(3): 417-26.

VanZuilen CD, Nickel RF, VanDijk TH, Reijngoud DJ. 1997. Xanthinuria in a family of Cavailier King Charles spaniels. *Veterinary Quarterly* **19**: 172-4.

Yarlagadda SG, Perazella MA. 2008. Drug-induced crystal nephropathy: an update. *Expert Opinion on Drug Safety* **7**(2): 147-58.

Chapter 5

Chapter 6
Proteinuria

Proteinuria can result from a variety of proteins excreted or lost into the urine. Albuminuria, the presence of albumin within urine, is the main contributor to overt proteinuria and is of the greatest clinical significance in dogs and cats. Detection of proteinuria includes both routine urinalysis and more advanced laboratory methods of urine testing. The ability to diagnose clinically relevant proteinuria is impacted by types of protein present, systemic disease, upper or lower urinary tract disease, and testing methodologies. This chapter reviews protein handling by the kidney, types of proteinuria, and diagnostic methods for identifying proteinuria.

Protein handling by the kidney

Normal urine contains little to no protein when compared to the amount presented to the kidney via renal blood flow. Renal protein handling is a balance of selective glomerular filtration and tubular reabsorption, both of which are intensely debated and researched topics in renal physiology and nephrology. Although much is known about glomerular filtration and tubular reabsorption, the amount of albumin that is normally able to pass into the filtrate as well as the impact of tubular reabsorption of albumin remain controversial topics. The relevance of the origin(s) of albuminuria impacts interpretation as a glomerular disease, a tubular disease, or a combination of both. In the coming years, additional research will likely further clarify the issue. While a comprehensive discussion of protein handling by the kidney is beyond the scope of this chapter, a brief synopsis of protein handling by the glomerulus and tubules is presented below. The reader is directed to any of a number of recent articles for greater understanding (Birn and Christensen 2006; Comper 2008; Comper et al. 2008, Haraldsson et al. 2008; Haraldsson and Jeansson 2009; Jarad and Miner 2009, Miner 2011, Nielsen and Christensen 2010; Osicka et al. 1997; Russo et al. 2002; Smithies 2003; Waller et al. 1989).

Practical Veterinary Urinalysis, First Edition. Carolyn Sink, Nicole Weinstein.
© 2012 John Wiley & Sons, Inc. Published 2012 by John Wiley & Sons, Inc.

Chapter 6

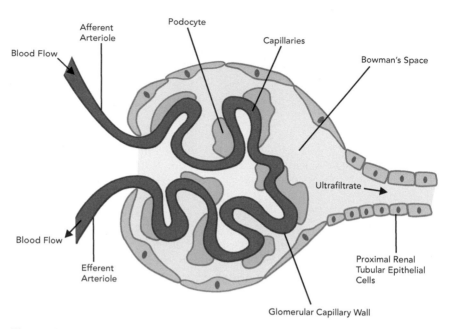

Figure 6.1 Glomerulus.

Glomerular filtration barrier

The anastamosed, twisted loops of capillaries contained within Bowman's capsule are the site of the glomerular filtration barrier (GFB) (Figure 6.1). As described in Chapter 1, the renal arterial blood supply feeds an afferent arteriole that supplies the glomerular capillary tuft; blood then exits via an efferent arteriole. The glomerular capillary wall (GCW) separates blood within the capillaries from the ultrafiltrate (in Bowman's space). The various layers and structural components of the GCW form the GFB (Abrahamson 1985; Comper and Russo 2009; Haraldsson and Jeansson 2009; Haraldsson et al. 2008; Kaneko 2008; Miner 2011). The actions of the GFB result in the formation of ultrafiltrate. The GCW is a complex, selective structure that determines the amount of protein, as well as various solutes, present in the ultrafiltrate. The exact composition and functions of the GCW are intensely researched. This research is rapidly altering the understanding of the selectivity of the filtration barrier (Abrahamson 1985, Comper 2009, Haraldsson and Jeansson 2009; Haraldsson et al. 2008; Miner 2011).

The basic components of the filtration barrier include an endothelial surface layer, a podocyte layer, and an intervening glomerular basement membrane (GBM), which is between the two cell layers. Endothelial cells line the internal aspect of the glomerular capillaries. These endothelial cells have pores (fenestrations) within the cells that allow for the passage of fluid. The endothelial cell surface displays a negatively charged glycocalyx, which is thought to be important in exclusion of albumin from the ultrafiltrate. Podocytes, also referred to as visceral epithelial cells, line the outside surface of the capillary (and so are present within Bowman's space and contact the ultrafiltrate). The podocytes encircle the outside of the glomerular capillaries via cytoplasmic projections known as foot processes, which abut one another. Between these interdigitating foot processes are filtration slits. A slit diaphragm, within a filtration slit, consists of many critical proteins that further determine selectivity of the GCW. The GBM is a shared intervening matrix, which is formed from the fusion of both the endothelial basement membrane and the visceral epithelial (podocyte) basement membrane (Abrahamson 1985; Jarad and Miner 2009; Miner 2011). The GBM contains specific molecules (i.e. glycoproteins, type IV collagen, and heparan sulfate proteoglycans) that are integral to the selectivity of the GFB. Abnormalities, either inherited or acquired, in any of the components or molecules within the various layers can result in proteinuria. Specific abnormalities of these components and molecules are extensively researched and are well described in human, rodent, and canine models of glomerular disease (Abrahamson 1985; Bader et al. 2005; Barker et al. 1990; Bonfanti et al. 2004; Futrakul et al. 2009; Jarad et al. 2006; Lees et al. 2002; Nabity et al. 2007; Zenker et al. 2004); etiology, prognosis, and treatment for these abnormalities are highly variable.

In the classical view of glomerular filtration, the GCW prevents larger proteins, greater than 70 kDa, from entering the ultrafiltrate. The interactions and specific attributes of the components of the GCW listed above collectively determine glomerular selectivity. In general terms, selectivity is a result of protein size and, to a lesser extent, electrical charge. Small proteins, of a low molecular weight (LMW), usually less than 40–60 kDa (Nabity et al. 2011), are able to pass through the GFB and enter the ultrafiltrate. If present in the capillary blood, these LMW proteins, including positive acute phase proteins (alpha and beta globulins that increase with inflammation), Bence-Jones protein, myoglobin, or hemoglobin (dimer), are able to pass into the ultrafiltrate. Larger proteins of a high molecular weight (HMW) are excluded due to their size (e.g. IgG, IgM, fibrinogen). Albumin, in the classical view, is, for the most part, unable to pass into the filtrate due to both size (at ~65 kD) and negative electrical charge. While size selectivity is generally an agreed-upon concept, continued debate concerns the role of electrical charge selectivity (Comper 2009; Comper et al. 2008; Haraldsson and Jeansson 2009).

Tubular reabsorption

Proximal renal tubular epithelial cells reabsorb, through the process of endocytosis, LMW proteins and albumin that pass through the GFB and enter the tubular fluid (Birn and Christensen 2006; Comper 2008; Comper 2009; Comper et al. 2008; Haraldsson and Jeansson 2009; Haraldsson et al. 2008; Nielsen and Christensen 2010; Saito et al. 2010). Endocytosis is mediated by

Chapter 6

the receptors megalin and cubilin (Nielsen and Christensen 2010; Saito et al. 2010). Lysosomal degradation of proteins within the epithelial cells follows (Birn and Christensen 2006; Comper 2008; Comper 2009; Comper et al. 2008; Haraldsson and Jeansson 2009; Haraldsson et al. 2008; Nielsen and Christensen 2010; Saito et al. 2010). With increasing amounts of albumin present in the renal tubular fluid, the limited reabsorption capacity is overwhelmed and albuminuria ensues. Increases in LMW proteins will also be detected in urine due to competition for megalin and cubilin binding sites (Nielsen and Christensen 2010; Vinge et al. 2010). Excessive albumin within the proximal renal tubule is hypothesized to cause inflammation and fibrosis given the increased demand on renal epithelial cells to process the excess proteins (Abbate et al. 2006; Birn and Christensen 2006; Futrakul et al. 2009; Ohse et al. 2006; Vinge et al. 2010). Although this has been demonstrated in *in vitro* studies, the role that an increased amount of albumin in the renal tubule plays in the pathogenesis of renal disease has yet to be fully realized. Medical treatments aimed at decreasing albuminuria seem to lessen the progression of renal disease (Hou et al. 2006). The relationship of albuminuria with prior renal damage, ongoing albumin-induced damage, or both, remains to be proven.

Significance of proteinuria

Normal urine contains only a small amount of protein that may not be detected by routine laboratory methods except when urine specific gravity (USG) is very high. Some of these proteins are synthesized by renal tubular epithelial cells, secreted into the tubular fluid, and excreted into the urine. Examples of these proteins include Tamm–Horsfall protein (in dogs), also known as uromodulin, immunoglobulin A, urokinase, and cauxin in cats (Biewenga et al. 1982; Nabity et al. 2011; Waller et al. 1989). Albumin is absent or present in non-detectable amounts (<1mg/dL).

In humans, even mild proteinuria, when due to albuminuria, is an independent risk factor for cardiovascular disease and is associated with a poorer outcome in patients with even only a mild decline in renal function (Hemmelgarn et al. 2010; Ruggenenti and Remuzzi 2006; Schrier 2007). In dogs and cats, the recognition of persistent albuminuria is evidence of underlying chronic kidney disease (CKD) (Grauer 2007; Jacob et al. 2005; Lees et al. 2005; Littman 2011). In addition to the standard diagnostic measures of renal disease, such as azotemia and inadequately concentrated urine, the presence of proteinuria, in both dogs and cats, is associated with decreased overall survival and can be an independent predictor of disease progression (Jacob et al. 2005; Kuwahara et al. 2006; Syme 2009; Syme et al. 2006; Vaden et al. 1997; Wehner et al. 2008). In dogs with chronic renal failure, a urine protein to creatinine (UPC) ratio of greater or equal to 1 had a greater risk of uremic crises and death when compared to dogs with a UPC of less than 1 (Jacob et al. 2005). Three separate studies in cats with renal disease revealed similar findings; an elevated UPC, even when only mildly increased (UPC > 0.2), was related to decreased survival (King et al. 2006; Kuwahara et al. 2006; Syme 2009; Syme et al. 2006). Proteinuria may be identified even in patients without overt renal disease. Over half of hospitalized dogs with various diseases were shown to have increased urine albumin concentrations (Grauer 2007; Whittemore et al. 2006). Another study demonstrated that diabetic dogs had higher urine albumin concentrations, and albuminuria alone was a significant predictor of hypertension (Struble et al. 1998).

Clinical assessment of proteinuria includes determining the type, the origin, the duration, and the severity of urine protein loss (Lees et al. 2005). The primary processes resulting in proteinuria include (1) increases in abnormal plasma proteins that enter into the tubular fluid and overwhelm resorptive capacity (overflow proteinuria); (2) altered or damaged GFB; (3) tubular injury or dysfunction resulting in a lack of protein resorption; and (4) tubular excretion. Proteinuria caused by albuminuria remains the most clinically relevant (Table 6.1).

Pathological proteinuria with urinary loss of albumin is caused by disease of the renal tubules, glomerulus, or a combination of both. Disease or damage to the renal interstitium can also result in proteinuria. Causes of pathological proteinuria due to tubular and/or glomerular disease are caused by a diverse and lengthy list of both inherited and acquired etiologies in dogs and cats (Grauer 2007; Littman 2011). Persistent proteinuria in younger animals should prompt consideration of an inherited abnormality in tubular reabsorption or glomerular function. Acquired causes of pathological proteinuria can be seen in any breed and is more common in dogs than cats (Littman 2011). Specific diagnoses may require biopsy with special processing and staining techniques as well as concurrent workup for an underlying systemic disease. Glomerulonephritis and amyloidosis are considered the most common causes of glomerular lesions in dogs and often result from infectious or immune-mediated diseases, although other etiologies are described (Grauer 2007; Grauer et al. 2002; Littman 2011). Drugs, such as glucocorticoids, can also result in glomerular changes and proteinuria (Waters et al. 1997). Interestingly, glucocorticoids are used to treat some types of glomerulonephritis. Several resources provide detailed information on both inherited and acquired causes as well as treatment options, when relevant (Grauer 2007; Lees et al. 2005; Littman 2011). In some cases, an inciting etiology may not be identified.

Laboratory diagnosis of proteinuria

The significance of proteinuria, specifically albuminuria, is undeniable, but definitive determination of proteinuria can present a diagnostic challenge. An active sediment, urine pH, method of collection have been implicated, to varying degrees, in altering protein levels in urine or impacting accurate measurement. Influence of collection methods and urinary tract inflammation

Table 6.1 Sources of urine protein

Prerenal or Preglomerular	*Overflow proteinuria*
	Various disease states can cause increased amounts of nonalbumin plasma protein(s) of mostly a low molecular weight (LMW). Small sized LMW proteins pass through the glomerular filtration barrier and exceed the resorptive capacity of the proximal renal tubule.
	Examples:
	  Acute-phase reactants due to inflammation and/or infection (e.g. pyometra, leptospirosis)
	  Hemoglobin from intravascular hemolysis
	  Myoglobin from rhabdomyolysis (severe muscle injury)
	  Immunoglobulin light chains (i.e., Bence Jones proteins) from underlying plasma cell or B cell neoplasia or infections

Renal	Proteinuria that results from abnormal handling by the kidney. It can be *functional* or *pathological*.
	Functional proteinuria reflects a response to a transient event (i.e., fever, seizure, and uncommonly, exercise, or is a result of altered renal protein handling.
	  The proteinuria is relatively **mild** and is **transient**, i.e., resolves following the resolution of the underlying condition.
	Pathological proteinuria (albuminuria) are due to altered structure or function of the kidneys:
	  1. *Glomerular*: Altered or damaged glomerular capillary wall
	  2. *Tubular:* Impaired tubular reabsorption of low molecular weight proteins +/- albumin
	  3. *Both* glomerular and tubular
	  4. *Interstitial*: Proteins enter the urine from peritubular capillaries (i.e., acute or chronic interstitial nephritis)

Post-renal	Proteinuria is a result of protein entering the urine at the renal pelvis (after urine has been formed) or further downstream.
	Post-renal proteinuria can be secondary to:
	  1. *Urinary* sources: proteins related to inflammation, hemorrhage, and/or neoplasia affecting the renal pelvis, ureters, urinary bladder, and urethra
	  2. *Extraurinary* sources: proteins originating from inflammation or hemorrhage of the genital tract and/or external genitalia and detected in urine collected from a voided or catheterized sample

Tubular secretion	Proteins are produced by renal tubular epithelial cells and secreted into tubular fluid. This type of proteinuria is mild and may only be detected in highly concentrated urine specimens.

Sources: Data from Bonfanti et al. (2004); Lees et al. (2005); Prober et al. (2010); Stockham and Scott (2008); Zaragosa et al. (2003, 2004).

and hemorrhage on diagnosis of proteinuria are addressed later in this chapter.

Methods of measurement of urine protein

Techniques for urine protein measurement vary in terms of sensitivity, specificity, and availability. Often, more than one test may be indicated. Methods include both routine measures and more advanced testing options:

Urine dipstick
Sulfosalicylic acid (SSA) precipitation
Urine protein to creatinine ratio
Microalbuminuria assays
Urine albumin to creatinine ratio

Urine dipstick

Urine dipsticks provide a semiquantitative measure of proteinuria but can be influenced by preanalytical, patient, and analytical variables. Also, urine dipstick measurement of protein may be of insufficient sensitivity to detect lower amounts of urine albumin, typically less than 30 mg/dL (300 g/L). Traditional interpretation of urine dipstick values is presented in Table 6.2. Urine protein dipstick methodology is covered in greater detail in Chapter 4, "Routine Urinalysis: Chemical Analysis."

The protein result on a urine dipstick generally should be evaluated in light of the patient's USG; a small amount of protein in dilute urine suggests more significant proteinuria when compared to the same amount in highly concentrated urine. Interpretation of urine dipstick protein is also influenced by the species of the patient. In general, the test is considered less reliable in cats due to frequent false-positive results (Lyon et al. 2010; Mardell and Sparkes 2006; Miyazaki et al. 2003, 2010; Moore et al. 1991). This increase in positive dipstick protein reactions is attributed to the excretion of non-albumin proteins, specifically cauxin (Miyazaki et al. 2003, 2010). Confirmatory tests are used to support a diagnosis of proteinuria or to grade proteinuria following

Chapter 6

Table 6.2 Interpretation of positive urine dipstick

Dipstick result	Interpretation
1+	30 mg/dL (0.3 g/L)
2+	100 mg/dL (1.0 g/L)
3+	300 mg/dL (3.0 g/L)
4+	1000 mg/dL (10.0 g/L)

Source: Data from Gregory (2003).

a positive dipstick result. Confirmatory tests include the SSA, UPC, or a microalbuminuria assay. Basic recommendations on interpretation, based on review of relevant literature, are provided below.

Sulfosalicylic acid

The SSA test, also known as the bumin test, is often used for confirmation of proteinuria following a positive result on a urine dipstick. The SSA test is a turbidometric assay and is traditionally considered a semiquantitative test. Chapter 4 also provides additional information on the SSA test. Equal quantities of urine supernatant and 5% SSA are mixed together in a tube, and degree of cloudiness (turbidity) is assessed. The acid denatures proteins present in the urine which causes precipitation of proteins and turbidity within the solution. The turbidity is then visually graded on a scale, 0 to 4. As little as 5 mg/dL of protein is reported to cause visual turbidity (Garner and Wiedmeyer 2007; Stockham and Scott 2008). To provide more quantitative results a set of standard solutions (0, 5, 10, 20, 30, 40, 50, 75, and 100 mg albumin/dL urine) (Cargille Modified Kinsbury-Clark Albumin Standards, Cargille Laboratories, Inc., Cedar Grove, NJ) can be used for comparison. The use of standards or spectrophotometric methods to assess turbidity, while providing more quantitative results is, admittedly, impractical in routine veterinary practice. The SSA test with visual inspection of turbidity is a relatively simple and reliable test, one that can be easily performed in practice.

General guidelines for interpretation in dogs and cats based on comparison to more advanced urine albumin testing methods have been recently proposed (Lyon et al. 2010). In dogs, positive results between the two tests should be similar to consider it a true positive when <2+ (Lyon et al. 2010). If either test result is ≥2+, the sample is likely positive for albumin in dogs (Lyon et al. 2010). Positive results necessitate additional testing for grading of proteinuria (Figure 6.2). In cats, urine dipstick and SSA both tend to result in a high number of false positives as previously mentioned. This may be a result of normally excreted non-albumin proteins (Miyazaki et al. 2003, 2010). For this reason, more specific testing for proteinuria, such as UPC or microalbuminuria assays, is recommended in cats (Lyon et al. 2010; Mardell and Sparkes 2006).

Urine protein to creatinine ratio

UPC has been the customary test used to confirm and/or stage proteinuria. The UPC, determined by measuring urine (total) protein and urine creatinine, is a quantitative measure of urine protein loss. It is most often measured at a reference laboratory, but some in-clinic options are available. Because albumin is the main protein in the urine, it is an estimate of urine albumin. More specific measures of urine albumin, however, are available and are discussed below. The gold standard in human medicine for urine protein excretion/loss, a 24-hour urine collection and protein measurement, is

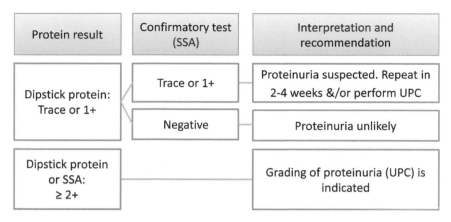

Figure 6.2 Interpretation of urine dipstick and SSA test in dogs. *Source:* Data from Lyon et al. (2010).

typically impractical in veterinary medicine. The UPC correlates well with the 24-hour collection as the creatinine measurement accounts for variations in urine volume throughout the day (Adams et al. 1992; Grauer et al. 1985; Lees et al. 2005; Monroe et al. 1989).

A consensus statement on proteinuria published in 2005 expanded on recommendations from the International Renal Interest Society (IRIS) and prior recommendations in the veterinary literature (www.iris-kidney.com). It provides guidelines for interpretation of UPC values in both dogs and cats. A value as low as 0.2 and greater is considered potentially clinically significant for proteinuria in both dogs and cats, especially if it is persistent and unrelated to prerenal or postrenal disease (Lees et al. 2005) (Table 6.3).

As mentioned earlier, UPC can be used both for confirmation or exclusion of significant proteinuria following a positive dipstick test as well as for grading overt proteinuria. When and if to perform a UPC is not always clear-cut. The recommendations of one study advise UPC testing in the following instances nces (Zatelli et al. 2010):

- Diagnosis proteinuria in dogs with a 1+ result and concurrent dilute urine (USG < 1.012)
- Grade proteinuria in dogs with a 2+ or greater urine protein result.

Additional testing was not indicated for dogs with 1+ or less proteinuria and a USG greater than 1.012 (Table 6.4).

Chapter 6

Table 6.3 Guidelines for interpretation of UPC in dogs and cats

Guidelines for interpretation of UPC in dogs

UPC	Interpretation
<0.2	Negative for proteinuria
≥0.2 to 0.4	Borderline proteinuria
≥0.5	Overt proteinuria

Guidelines for interpretation of UPC in cats

UPC	Interpretation
<0.2	Negative for proteinuria
≥0.2 to 0.3	Borderline proteinuria
≥0.4	Overt proteinuria

Source: Data from Lees et al. (2005).

Table 6.4 Suggested interpretation of dipstick and USG results

	Dipstick test results		
USG	0 (0 mg/dL)	1+ (30 mg/dL)	2+ (≥100 mg/dL)
≤1.012	NP	UPC ratio	UPC ratio
>1.012; <1.030	NP	NP	UPC ratio
≥1.030	NP	NP	UPC ratio

NP, nonproteinuric, quantification of urine protein not required.
Source: Data from Zatelli et al. (2010).

UPC values may exhibit enough day-to-day variation in a patient to risk misdiagnosis (Nabity et al. 2007). Ideally, urine should be sampled over several days, using the same sampling method, to determine a patient's UPC (Fernandes et al. 2005; Nabity et al. 2007). This may not be an option for all patients given the added expense of submitting multiple urine samples for UPC determination. Pooling urine samples of equal volumes from the same dog over 3 days was demonstrated to be a reliable and cost-effective alternative for UPC testing over multiple days (Levine et al. 2010). Additionally, once a baseline UPC is determined for a patient, the same methodology (i.e. analyzer and/or reference laboratory) should be used to monitor the patient's UPC (Fernandes et al. 2005).

Chapter 6

Table 6.5 Multistix PRO dipstick–protein interpretation

Test pad	Protein–low	Protein–high[a]	Interpretation
	Color change	No color change	15 mg/dL
	Color change	Color change	≥30-300 mg/dL
	No color change	No color change	Negative[b]

[a] Similar methodology to routine dipstick protein methodology; includes 30, 100, or 300 mg/dL.
[b] Protein concentration is below the sensitivity of the "protein–low" reagent pad.

In-clinic UPC dipstick

A special urine dipstick test is available for in-clinic determination of UPC; it was demonstrated to be useful in dogs, but not in cats (Welles et al. 2006).

Multistix PRO (Bayer Corporation, Elkhart, IN)

The Multistix PRO is similar to a routine urine dipstick with the addition of a specific test pad for measurement of urine creatinine and two levels of urine protein measurement. Reading of the test pad is by either visual examination or by a Clinitek 50 analyzer (Bayer Corporation, Tarrytown, NY). For visual determination, results on the Multistix PRO dipstick are compared to a color chart similar to routine urine dipsticks. The higher protein result is reported of the two pads (protein–low or protein–high); if both are negative, the results are "negative" (Strasinger and DiLorenzo 2008) (Table 6.5). The UPC value determined by the analyzer (denoted P:C) gives a result in mg/g (divide protein value by 0.1 g creatinine/dL) and "normal" or "abnormal" interpretation:

Normal: <150 mg protein/g creatinine
Abnormal: 150, 300, and >500 mg protein/g creatinine.

A chart, provided by the manufacturer, assists in interpretation. A UPC can be calculated manually using the protein and creatinine values provided by the dipstick (or analyzer): divide the protein value (mg protein/dL) by the creatinine value (mg creatinine/dL). When compared to quantitative biochemical determination of UPC, a negative protein result using the Multistix PRO dipstick resulted in a very high likelihood (97%) the patient is truly negative for clinically significant proteinuria (Welles et al. 2006). Evaluation of UPC values from both manual calculation and machine calculation, using the Clinitek instrument, were recommended for confirmation and interpretation of positive results (Welles et al. 2006). The Multistix PRO is not recommended for determination of UPC in cats (Welles et al. 2006).

Additional considerations for UPC

UPC measurement may not detect very low levels of albuminuria, which may reflect early renal disease. The use of UPC as a screening test has been

Chapter 6

questioned, and testing for microalbuminuria using a species-specifc antibody to albumin may offer greater sensitivity in both dogs and cats (Garner and Wiedmeyer 2007; Langston 2004; Lyon et al. 2010; Syme et al. 2006). Grading of overt proteinuria and recommendations for treatment or management of proteinuria rely on interpretation of UPC numerical results, which support its continued use.

Microalbuminuria assays

Microalbuminuria is the presence of urine albumin that is not detected by a standard urine dipstick, typically lower than 20–30 mg/dL (<200–300 mg/L) (Futrakul et al. 2009; Ruggenenti and Remuzzi 2006; Vaden et al. 2001). Microalbuminuria has been defined as an albumin concentration within 1.0 and 30.0 mg/dL (10–300 mg/L) in urine normalized to a specific gravity of 1.010 (Gentilini et al. 2005; Murgier et al. 2009; Vaden 2003).

In humans, the presence of microalbuminuria is associated with increased risk of mortality, progression to kidney failure, and myocardial infarction (Futrakul et al. 2009; Hemmelgarn et al. 2010). Microalbuminuria has been shown to be more prevalent in older dogs when compared to younger dogs and, not surprisingly, in dogs with urinary tract disease, neoplasia, infectious, inflammatory, or immune-mediated diseases, and other disease types (ERD product insert 2003; Jensen et al. 2001, 2011; Pressler et al. 2001; Radecki et al. 2003; Whittemore et al. 2006). Over half of dogs with microalbuminuria, but not proteinuria, were found to have an "underlying systemic disease" (Whittemore et al. 2003). Microalbuminuria is also associated with underlying systemic disease in cats, including urinary tract disease (Whittemore et al. 2007). Earlier identification of renal disease, specifically albuminuria below the limit of standard detection methods, allows for clinical intervention which may slow disease progression (Vaden 2003). Several tests are available for screening of patients for microalbuminuria.

Laboratory analysis of microalbuminuria

In-clinic tests include the Early Renal Detection (ERD)-Health Screen, Clinitek Microalbumin reagent strip (Clinitek Microalbumin, Bayer Corporation, Elkhart, IN), and the micral test strip. The latter two strips use a monoclonal antibody to human albumin while the ERD-Health Screen uses a species-specific antibody.

ERD or ERD-Health Screen® (Heska, Fort Collins, CO): Canine or feline specific

Methodology
ERD-Health Screen is a semiquantitative immunoassay. The testing pad utilizes a species-specific (canine or feline) monoclonal antibody against albumin. The test identifies urine samples containing greater than 1mg/dL of albumin

(ERD product insert 2003; Garner and Wiedmeyer 2007). Collected urine is diluted, in accordance with the provided procedure, to a specific gravity of 1.010; this helps to standardize the measurement across a range of urine concentrating ability (ERD product insert 2003; Langston 2004; Murgier et al. 2009). This type of standardization is similar to comparison to urine creatinine in UPC or urine albumin to creatinine (UAC) ratios and yields comparable prognostic information (Syme and Elliot 2005). After the test device with pad is inserted into the urine, colored lines develop and indicate if the albumin concentration is less than 1mg/dL (negative) or greater than 1mg/dL (positive). Positive reactions are further classified as low, medium, high, or very high based on intensity of the reaction; grading is somewhat subjective (Mardell and Sparkes 2006).

Conclusion

The ERD-Health Screen has been shown to be highly correlated to UPC and may offer greater sensitivity for detection of low levels of albuminuria than other in-clinic tests (Garner and Wiedmeyer 2007; Lyon et al. 2010; Mardell and Sparkes 2006). Given the increased likelihood of false-positive urine dipstick protein reactions in cats, this assay may be used as an in-clinic option to confirm or identify proteinuria. It is less useful for overt proteinuria.

Clinitek Microalbumin reagent strip

Methodology

The Clinitek Microalbumin reagent strip uses an antibody-impregnated pad that binds to human albumin. The reagent strip uses two reaction pads that allow, with the use of color comparison charts, a visual estimate of albumin and creatinine concentrations; alternatively, results can be evaluated with the use of a Clinitek analyzer (Bayer).

Conclusion

Clinitek Microalbumin reagent strips demonstrate low sensitivity. This makes them a poor screening test in dogs for detection of microalbuminuria (Pressler et al. 2002).

Micral (Roche Diagnostics Corporation, IN)

Methodology

Micral test strips rely upon antibody-impregnated pads that bind to human albumin. The series of reagent pads produce an antibody–enzyme complex that reacts with a single color-substrate pad. The final color on the pad is then compared to a reference chart.

Conclusion

This test should not be used as a screening test in dogs for detection of microalbuminuria (Pressler et al. 2002).

Chapter 6

Urine albumin or urine albumin to creatinine ratio

Tests for urine albumin or UAC ratio have been developed for both detection of albuminuria as well as quantitative measurement of albumin in cerebro-spinal fluid (Gentilini et al. 2005; Kuwahara et al. 2008). While these tests would offer greater sensitivity and specificity for albumin detection when compared to traditional in-clinic tests (i.e. urine dipstick or SSA test), the UAC provides similar information to the UPC. UAC results are also not directly comparable to UPC, and recommendations for diagnosis and treatment of proteinuria are currently based on UPC ranges. Currently, both urine albumin tests and UAC measurement are limited to research and few reference laboratories.

Recommendations regarding diagnosis of proteinuria

Current recommendations regarding proteinuria are based on UPC values, presence or absence of microalbuminuria, and other clinical or laboratory findings pertinent to the patient such as concurrent azotemia (Lees et al. 2005). Recommendations include when to monitor for persistent or worsening proteinuria, when to investigate an underlying cause, and when to medically intervene. Figure 6.3 provides a brief summary of the first phase, monitoring proteinuria (Lees et al. 2005). While the latter two are beyond the scope of this chapter, several resources provide detailed information for both diagnostic and treatment options in patients with persistent proteinuria (Grauer 2007; Lees et al. 2005; Littman 2011; www.iris-kidney.com).

Additional considerations for proteinuria

Method of collection

Collection type has been previously reported to impact UPC in male dogs; recently, however, it was demonstrated either free catch or cystocentesis result in equivalent UPC values (Barsanti and Finco 1979; Beatrice et al. 2010).

Semen contamination of urine

Semen-containing urine samples may result in a false-positive urine dipstick protein result (Prober et al. 2010).

Urinary tract inflammation and hemorrhage

Caution in interpretation of a urine dipstick result is suggested when inflammation and/or hemorrhage within the urinary tract is present. In a patient with an active urinary sediment, a positive protein result should not be attributed entirely to postrenal inflammation or hemorrhage. Although increases

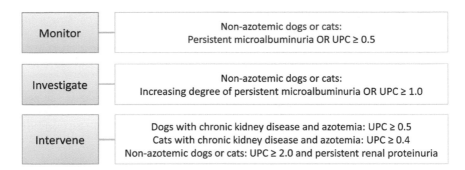

Figure 6.3 Consensus recommendations for proteinuria.
Sources: Data from Grauer et al. (1985); Lees et al. (2005); Littman (2011);
http://www.iris-kidney.com

in urine albumin can result from macroscopic hematuria with or without
pyuria, the UPC does not often increase (Vaden et al. 2004). Also, there is
poor correlation between UPC and degree of hematuria or pyuria (Bagley et
al. 1991). Both have been shown to contribute minimally to proteinuria or UPC
in dog. Even in the presence of macroscopic hematuria and in most cases of
pyuria, UPC remains less than 0.5 (Vaden et al. 2004).

References

Abbate M, Zoja C, Remuzzi G. 2006. How does proteinuria cause progressive renal
damage? *Journal of the American Society of Nephrology* **17**: 2974-84.

Abrahamson DR. 1985. Origin of the glomerular basement membrane visualized
after *in vivo* labeling of laminin in newborn rat kidneys. *Journal of Cell Biology*
100: 1988-2000.

Adams LG, Polzin DJ, Osborne CA, O'Brien TD. 1992. Correlation of urine protein/
creatinine ratio and twenty-four-hour urinary protein excretion in normal cats
and cats with surgically induced chronic renal failure. *Journal of Veterinary
Internal Medicine* **6**(3): 6-40.

Bader BL, Smyth N, Nedbal S, Miosge N, Baranowsky A, Mokkapati S, Murshed M,
Nischt R. 2005. Compound genetic ablation of nidogen 1 and 2 causes basement
membrane defects and perinatal lethality in mice. *Molecular and Cell Biology*
25: 6846-56.

Bagley RS, Center SA, Lewis RM. 1991. The effect of experimental cystitis and
iatrogenic blood contamination on the urine protein/creatinine ratio in the dog.
Journal of Veterinary Internal Medicine **5**: 66-70.

Barker DF, Hostikka SL, Zhou J, Chow LT, Oliphant AR, Gerken SC, Gregory MC,
Skolnick MH, Atkin CL, Tryggvason K. 1990. Identification of mutations in the
COL4A5 collagen gene in Alport syndrome. *Science* **248**: 1224-7.

Barsanti JA, Finco DR. 1979. Protein concentration in urine of normal dogs. *American Journal of Veterinary Research* **40**: 1583-8.

Beatrice L, Nizi F, Callegari D, Paltrinieri S, Zini E, D'Ippolito P, Zatelli A. 2010.
Comparison of urine protein-to-creatinine ratio in urine samples collected by

cystocentesis versus free catch in dogs. *Journal of the American Veterinary Medical Association* **236**(11): 1221-4.

Biewenga WJ, Gruys E, Hendicks HJ. 1982. Urinary protein loss in the dog. Nephrological study of 29 dogs without signs of renal disease. *Research in Veterinary Science* **33**: 366-74.

Birn H, Christensen EI. 2006. Renal albumin absorption in physiology and pathology. *Kidney International* **69**: 440-9.

Bonfanti U, Zini E, Minetti E, Zatelli A. 2004. Free light-chain proteinuria and normal renal histopathology and function in 11 dogs exposed to *Leishmania infantum*, *Ehrlichia canis*, and *Babesia canis*. *Journal of Veterinary Internal Medicine* **18**(5): 618-24.

Comper WD. 2008. Resolved: normal glomeruli filter nephrotic levels of albumin. *Journal of the American Society of Nephrology* **19**: 427-32.

Comper WD, Hilliard LM, Nikolic-Paterson DJ, Russo LM. 2008. Disease-dependent mechanisms of albumuria. *American Journal Physiology. Renal Physiology* **295**: F1589-F1600.

Comper WD, Russo LM. 2009. The glomerular filter: an imperfect barrier is required for perfect renal function. *Current Opinion in Nephrology and Hypertension* **18**(4): 336-42.

ERD-HealthScreen Canine and Feline Urine Tests Product Insert. 2003. Heska Corp, Loveland, CO.

Fernandes P, Kahn M, Yang V, Weilbacher A. 2005. Comparison of methods used for determining urine protein-to-creatinine ratio in dogs and cats [abstract]. *Journal of Veterinary Internal Medicine* **19**(3): 431.

Futrakul N, Sridama V, Futrakul P. 2009. Microalbuminuria–a biomarker of renal microvascular disease. *Renal Failure* **31**(2): 140-3.

Garner BC, Wiedmeyer CE. 2007. Comparison of a semiquantitative point-of-care assay for the detection of canine microalbuminuria with routine semiquantitative methods for proteinuria. *Veterinary Clinical Pathology* **36**: 240-4.

Gentilini F, Dondi F, Mastrorilli C, Giunti M, Calzolari C, Gandini G, Mancini D, Bergamini PF. 2005. Validation of a human immunoturbidometric assay to measure canine albumin in urine and cerebrospinal fluid. *Journal of Veterinary Diagnostic Investigation* **17**: 179-83.

Grauer GF. 2007. Measurement, interpretation, and implications of proteinuria and albuminuria. *Veterinary Clinics Small Animal Practice* **37**: 283-95.

Grauer GF, Thomas CB, Eicker SW. 1985. Estimation of quantitative proteinuria in the dog, using the urine protein-to-creatinine ratio from a random, voided sample. *American Journal of Veterinary Research* **46**(10): 2116-9.

Grauer GF, Oberhauser EB, Basaraba RJ, Lappin MR, Simpson DF, Jensen WA. 2002. Development of microalbuminuria in dogs with heartworm disease. *Journal of Veterinary Internal Medicine* **16**: 352.

Gregory CR. 2003. Urinary system. In *Duncan & Prasse's Veterinary Laboratory Medicine Clinical Pathology*, 4th ed. Latimer KS, Mahaffe EA, Prasse KW, eds., pp. 231-59. Ames, IA: Iowa State Press.

Haraldsson B, Jeansson M. 2009. Glomerular filtration barrier. *Current Opinion in Nephrology and Hypertension* **18**: 331-5.

Haraldsson B, Nystrom J, Deen WM. 2008. Properties of the glomerular barrier and mechanisms of proteinuria. *Physiological Reviews* **88**: 451-87.

Hemmelgarn BR, Manns BJ, Lloyd A, James MT, Klarenback S, Quinn RR, Wiebe N, Tonelli M. 2010. Relation between kidney function, proteinuria, and adverse outcomes. *Journal of the American Medical Association* **303**(5): 423-9.

Hou FF, Zhang X, Zhang GH, Xie D, Chen PY, Zhang WR, Jiang JP, Liang M, Wang GB, Liu ZR, Geng RW. 2006. Efficacy and safety of benazepril for advanced chronic renal insufficiency. *New England Journal of Medicine* **354**: 131–40.

Jacob F, Polzin DJ, Osborne CA et al. 2005. Evaluation of the association between initial proteinuria and morbidity rate or death in dogs with naturally occurring chronic renal failure. *Journal of the American Veterinary Medical Association* **226**: 393–400.

Jarad G, Miner JH. 2009. Update on the glomerular filtration barrier. *Current Opinion in Nephrology and Hypertension* **18**(3): 226–32.

Jarad G, Cunningham J, Shaw AS, Miner JH. 2006. Proteinuria precedes podocyte abnormalities in Lamb2-/- mice, implicating the glomerular basement membrane as an albumin barrier. *Journal of Clinical Investigation* **116**: 2272–9.

Jensen WA, Grauer GF, Andrews J, Simpson D. 2001. Prevalence of microalbuminuria in dogs [abstract]. *Journal of Veterinary Internal Medicine* **15**: 300.

Jensen WA, Cleland WP, Donnelly R et al. 2011. New data: identification of underlying disease in dogs that test positive with the E.R.D.-HealthScreen canine urine test. Available at: www.heska.com/Documents/RenalHealthScreen/erd_data572.aspx.

Kaneko JJ. 2008. Kidney function and damage. In *Clinical Biochemistry of Domestic Animals*, 6th ed. Kaneko JJ, Harvey JW, Bruss ML, eds., pp. 485–528. Burlington, VT: Elsevier Inc.

King JN, Tasker S, Gunn-Moore DA, Strehlau G. BENRIC Study Group. 2006. Prognostic factors in cats with chronic kidney disease. *Journal of Veterinary Internal Medicine* **20**: 1054–64.

Kuwahara Y, Ohba Y, Kitoh K, Kuwahara N, Kitagawa H. 2006. Association of laboratory data and death within one month in cats with chronic renal failure. *The Journal of Small Animal Practice* **47**: 446–50.

Kuwahara Y, Nishii N, Takasu M, Ohba Y, Maeda S, Kitawaga H. 2008. Use of urine albumin/creatinine ratio for estimation of proteinuria in cats and dogs. *Journal of Veterinary Medical Science* **70**(8): 865–7.

Langston C. 2004. Microalbuminuria in cats. *Journal of the American Animal Hospital Association* **40**: 251–4.

Lees GE et al. 2002. Persistent albuminuria precedes onset of overt proteinuria in male dogs with X-linked hereditary nephropathy. *Journal of Veterinary Internal Medicine* **16**: 353.

Lees GE, Brown SA, Elliott J et al. 2005. Assessment and management of proteinuria in dogs and cats: 2004 ACVIM Forum Consensus Statement (small animal). *Journal of Veterinary Internal Medicine* **19**: 377–85.

LeVine DM, Zhang D, Harris T, Vaden SL. 2010. The use of pooled vs serial urine samples to measure urine protein: creatinine ratios. *Veterinary Clinical Pathology* **39**(1): 53–6.

Littman MP. 2011. Protein-losing nephropathy in small animals. *Veterinary Clinics of North America. Small Animal Practice* **41**: 31–62.

Lyon SD, Sanderson MW, Vaden SL, Lappin MR, Jensen WA, Grauer GF. 2010. Comparison of urine dipstick, sulfosalicylic acid, urine protein-to-creatinine ratio, and species-specific ELISA methods for detection of albumin in urine samples of cats and dogs. *Journal of the American Veterinary Medical Association* **236**: 874–9.

Mardell EJ, Sparkes AH. 2006. Evaluation of a commercial in-house test kit for the semi-quantitative assessment of microalbuminuria in cats. *Journal of Feline Medicine and Surgery* **8**: 269–78.

Chapter 6

Miner JH. 2011. Glomerular basement membrane composition and the filtration barrier. *Pediatric Nephrology* **9**: 1413-7. Epub February 15, 2011.

Miyazaki M, Kamiie K, Soeta S, Taira H, Yamashita T. 2003. Molecular cloning and characterization of a novel carboxylesterase-like protein that is physiologically present at high concentrations in the urine of domestic cats (*Felis catus*). *Biochemical Journal* **370**(Pt 1): 101-10.

Miyazaki M, Fujiwara K, Suzuta Y, Hobuko W, Taira H, Suzuki A, Yamashita T. 2010. Screening for proteinuria in cats using a conventional dipstick test after removal of cauxin from urine with a *Lens culinaris* agglutinin lectin tip. *The Veterinary Journal*. Available at: www.sciencedirect.com/science/article/pii/S1090023310002844.

Monroe WE, Davenport DJ, Saunders GK. 1989. Twenty-four hour urinary protein loss in healthy cats and the urinary protein-creatinine ratio as an estimate. *American Journal of Veterinary Research*. **50**(11): 1906-9.

Moore FM, Brum SL, Brown L. 1991. Urine protein determination in dogs and cats: comparison of dipstick and sulfosalicylic acid procedures. *Veterinary Clinical Pathology* **20**(4): 95-7.

Murgier P, Jakins A, Bexfield N, Archer J. 2009. Comparison of semiquantitative test strips, urine protein electrophoresis, and an immunoturbidimetric assay for measuring microalbuminuria in dogs. *Veterinary Clinical Pathology* **38**(4): 485-92.

Nabity MB, Boggess MM, Kashtan CE, Lees GE. 2007. Day-to-day variation of the urine protein : creatinine ratio in female dogs with stable glomerular proteinuria caused by x-linked hereditary nephropathy. *Journal of Veterinary Internal Medicine* **21**: 425-30.

Nabity MB, Lees GE, Dangott LJ, Cianciolo R, Suchodolski JS, Steiner JM. 2011. Proteomic analysis of urine from male dogs during early stages of tubulointerstitial injury in a canine model of progressive glomerular disease. *Veterinary Clinical Pathology* **40**(2): 222-36.

Nielsen R, Christensen EI. 2010. Proteinuria and events beyond the slit. *Pediatric Nephrology* **25**: 813-22.

Ohse T, Inagi R, Tanaka T, Ota T, Miyata T, Kojima I, Ingelfinger JR, Ogawa S, Fujita T, Nangaku M. 2006. Albumin induces endoplasmic reticulum stress and apoptosis in renal proximal tubular cells. *Kidney International* **70**: 1447-55.

Osicka TM, Panagiotopoulos S, Jerums G, Comper WD. 1997. Fractional clearance of albumin is influenced by its degradation during renal passage. *Clinical Science (London)* **93**: 557-64.

Pressler BM, Vaden SL, Jensen WA, Simpson D. 2001. Prevalence of microalbuminuria in dogs evaluated at a referral veterinary hospital [abstract]. *Journal of Veterinary Internal Medicine* **15**: 300.

Pressler BM, Vaden SL, Jensen WA, Simpson D. 2002. Detection of canine microalbuminuria using a semiquantitative test strips designed for use with human urine. *Veterinary Clinical Pathology* **31**: 56-60.

Prober LG, Johnson CA, Olivier NB, Thomas JS. 2010. Effect of semen in urine specimens on urine protein concentration determined by means of dipstick analysis. *American Journal of Veterinary Research* **71**: 288-92.

Radecki S, Donnely R, Jensen WA, et al. 2003. Effect of age and breed on the prevalence of microalbuminuria in dogs (abstract). *Journal of Veterinary Internal Medicine* **17**: 406.

Ruggenenti P, Remuzzi G. 2006. Time to abandon microalbuminuria? *Kidney International* **70**: 1214-22.

Russo LM, Bakris GL, Comper WD. 2002. Renal handling of albumin: a critical review of basic concepts and perspective. *American Journal of Kidney Disease* **39**: 899–919.

Saito A, Sato H, Iino N, Takeda T. 2010. Molecular mechanisms of receptor-mediated endocytosis in the renal proximal tubular epithelium. *Journal of Biomedicine and Biotechnology* **2010**: 1–7.

Schrier RW. 2007. Laboratory evaluation of kidney function. In *Diseases of the Kidney and Urinary Tract*, vol. 1, 8th ed. Schrier RW, ed., pp. 299–336. Philadelphia: Lippincott Williams and Wilkins.

Smithies O. 2003. Why the kidney glomerulus does not clog: a gel permeation/diffusion hypothesis of renal function. *Proceedings of the National Academy of Sciences of the United States of America* **100**(7): 4108–13.

Stockham SL, Scott MA. 2008. Urinary system. In *Fundamentals of Veterinary Clinical Pathology*, 2nd ed. Stockham SL, Scott MA, eds., pp. 415–94. Ames, IA: Blackwell Publishing.

Strasinger SK, DiLorenzo MS. 2008. Physical examination of urine. In *Urinalysis and Body Fluids*, 5th ed. Strasinger SK, DiLorenzo MS, eds., pp. 41–51. Philadelphia: FA Davis Company.

Struble AL, Feldman EC, Nelson RW, Kass PH. 1998. Systemic hypertension and proteinuria in dogs with diabetes mellitus. *Journal of the American Veterinary Medical Association* **213**(6): 822–5.

Syme HM. 2009. Proteinuria in cats: prognostic marker or mediator? *Journal of Feline Medicine and Surgery* **11**(3): 211–8.

Syme HM, Elliot J. 2005. Comparison of urinary albumin excretion normalized by creatinine concentration or urine specific gravity. *Journal of Veterinary Internal Medicine* **19**(3): 466.

Syme HM, Markwell PJ, Pfeiffer D, Elliot J. 2006. Survival of cats with naturally occurring chronic renal failure is related to severity of proteinuria. *Journal of Veterinary Internal Medicine* **20**: 528–35.

Vaden S. 2003. Microalbuminuria: what is it and how do I interpret it? *Proceedings, 21st American College of Veterinary Internal Medicine Forum*.

Vaden SL, Levine J, Breitschwerdt EB. 1997. A retrospective case-control of acute renal failure in 99 dogs. *Journal of Veterinary Internal Medicine* **11**(2): 58–64.

Vaden SL et al. 2001. Longitudinal study of microalbuminuria in soft-coated Wheaten Terriers. *Journal of Veterinary Internal Medicine* **15**: 300.

Vaden SL, Pressler BM, Lappin MR, Jensen WA. 2004. Effects of urinary tract inflammation and sample blood contamination on urine albumin and total protein concentrations in canine urine samples. *Veterinary Clinical Pathology* **33**: 14–9.

Vinge L, Lees GE, Nielsen R, Kashtan CE, Bahr A, Christensen EI. 2010. The effect of progressive glomerular disease on megalin-mediated endocytosis in the kidney. *Nephrology, Dialysis, Transplantation* **25**(8): 2458–67. Epub March 2, 2010.

Waller KV, Ward MW, Mahan JD, Wismatt DK. 1989. Current concepts in proteinuria. *Clinical Chemistry* **35**: 5.

Waters CB, Adams LG, Scott-Moncrieff JC, DeNicola DB, Snyder PW, White MR, Gasparini M. 1997. Effects of glucocorticoid therapy on urine protein-to-creatinine ratios and renal morphology in dogs. *Journal of Veterinary Internal Medicine* **11**: 172–7.

Wehner A, Hartmann K, Hirschberger J. 2008. Associations between proteinuria, systemic hypertension and glomerular filtration rate in dogs with renal and non-renal diseases. *The Veterinary Record* **162**(5): 141–7.

Chapter 6

Welles EG, Whatley EM, Hall AS, Wright JC. 2006. Comparison of Multistix PRO dipsticks with other biochemical assays for determining urine protein (UP), urine creatinine (UC), and UP : UC ratio in dogs and cats. *Veterinary Clinical Pathology* **35**(1): 31-6.

Whittemore JC, Jensen WA, Prause L, Radecki S, Gill V, Lappin MR. 2003. Comparison of microalbuminuria, urine protein dipstick, and urine protein creatinine ratio results in clinically ill dogs [abstract]. *Journal of Veterinary Internal Medicine* **17**: 437.

Whittemore JC, Gill VL, Jensen WA, Radecki SV, Lappin MR. 2006. Evaluation of the association between microalbuminuria and the urine albumin creatinine ratio and systemic disease in dogs. *Journal of the American Veterinary Medical Association* **229**: 958-63.

Whittemore JC, Miyoshi Z, Jensen WA, Radecki SV, Lappin MR. 2007. Association of microalbuminuria and the urine albumin-to-creatinine ratio with systemic disease in cats. *Journal of the American Veterinary Medical Association* **230**(8): 1165-9.

Zaragosa C, Barrera R, Centeno F, Tapia JA, Mane MC. 2003. Characterization of renal damage in canine leptospirosis by sodium dodecyl sulphate-polyacrylamide gel electrophoresis (SDS-PAGE) and Western blotting of the urinary proteins. *Journal of Comparative Pathology* **129**(2-3): 169-78.

Zaragosa C, Barrera R, Centeno F, Tapia JA, Mane MC. 2004. Canine pyometra: a study of the urinary proteins by SDS-PAGE and Western blot. *Theriogenology* **61**(7): 1259-72.

Zatelli A, Paltrinieri S, Nizi F, Roura X, Zini E. 2010. Evaluation of a urine dipstick test for confirmation or exclusion of proteinuria in dogs. *American Journal of Veterinary Research* **71**(2): 235-40.

zZenker M, Tralau T, Lennert T, Pitz S, Mark K, Madlon H, Dotsch J, Reis A, Muntefering H, Neumann LM. 2004. Congenital nephrosis, mesangial sclerosis, and distinct eye abnormalities with microcoria: an autosomal recessive syndrome. *American Journal of Medical Genetics. Part A* **130**: 138-45.

Chapter 6

Webliography

www.iris-kidney.com Website of the International Renal Interest Society (IRIS), provides information on diagnosis and treatment of kidney disease in dogs and cats.

Chapter 7
Advanced Diagnostics

Routine urinalysis, when performed in conjunction with a complete blood count and chemistry panel, provides information about patient health and can identify underlying disease, if present. Urinalysis and the standard measures of renal function, blood urea nitrogen (BUN) and creatinine, may not always be abnormal in cases of acute or subclinical renal disease. Monitoring the magnitude of injury and progression of renal disease is a useful prognostic and therapeutic tool but may require tests of greater sensitivity and specificity. An abnormal urinalysis itself may necessitate additional testing (e.g. bacterial culture, urine cytology) to further characterize any abnormalities detected.

As described in Chapter 1, inadequate concentrating ability and azotemia typically develop only after greater than 66-75% of functioning nephrons are impaired or lost (Stockham and Scott 2008). Evidence of tubular injury in the form of cellular, granular, and/or waxy casts may not be present in all cases of acute renal disease (Vaden et al. 1997). A variety of tests have been described that more accurately assess renal function, monitor for renal injury, and diagnose specific diseases. Many of these tests remain under investigation or require further standardization but may be more widely available and understood in the future. The following is not an exhaustive list of options; the aim is to provide the reader with additional resources and test methodologies for diagnostic consideration.

Detection of bacteriuria versus diagnosis of urinary tract infection

Diagnosis of urinary tract infections (UTIs) most often utilizes evaluation of urine sediment to identify pyuria, the presence of neutrophils within urine, and bacteriuria as reliance on biochemical methods (i.e. urine dipstick) is unreliable in veterinary medicine (Klausner et al. 1976). Sediment evaluation is a routine component of urinalysis and is described in Chapter 5, with representative images provided. Bacterial culture can also be used for both identification and characterization of bacterial population(s) present. The presence of bacteria within a urine sample is not equivalent to diagnosis of UTI. A diagnosis of the latter is more likely when bacteria are identified upon sediment examination of an aseptically obtained sample and/or in samples with concurrent pyuria (>3–5 WBCs/hpf in cystocentesis-collected samples or >5 WBCs/HPF in samples obtained by free catch or catheter) (Bartges 2004).

Stained air-dried sediment smears

Detection of bacteriuria via sediment examination can be challenging in some instances despite clinical suspicion of a UTI. This is especially true in dilute urine samples. Submission of urine for bacterial culture, while a sensitive test, may not be the most cost-effective if the index of suspicion for a UTI is low (Tivapasi et al. 2009). Microscopic evaluation of an air-dried urine sediment smear offers greater sensitivity and specificity in detection of bacteriuria compared to evaluation of unstained urine sediment (Swenson et al. 2004) (Figure 7.1a,b).

Procedure:
1. Centrifuge urine (see Chapter 5 for the full procedure).
2. Remove a small drop of urine sediment and place on a clean glass slide. A coverslip or pipette tip can be used to gently spread the sediment on the slide to make a thin preparation.
3. Allow slide with sediment to air dry.
4. Stain slide (Diff-Quik, Dade Behring, Inc., Newark, NJ).
5. Raise the condenser of the microscope to just under the stage to decrease contrast (the stain provides the necessary contrast).
6. Evaluate for bacteria, leukocytes, and other elements under 100× oil or place a drop of oil, followed by a coverslip and evaluate under 40×.

Bacterial culture of urine

Ideally, bacterial culture should be performed on urine samples collected in a sterile manner, typically by cystocentesis. A veterinary reference laboratory most often performs bacterial culture of urine, although some larger in-clinic laboratories may offer this service. Quantitative bacterial cultures are considered the gold standard as both numbers and type(s) of bacterial organisms are determined. Samples should be contained within a sterile container and kept refrigerated until processed as bacteria rapidly multiply at room temperature.

Chapter 7

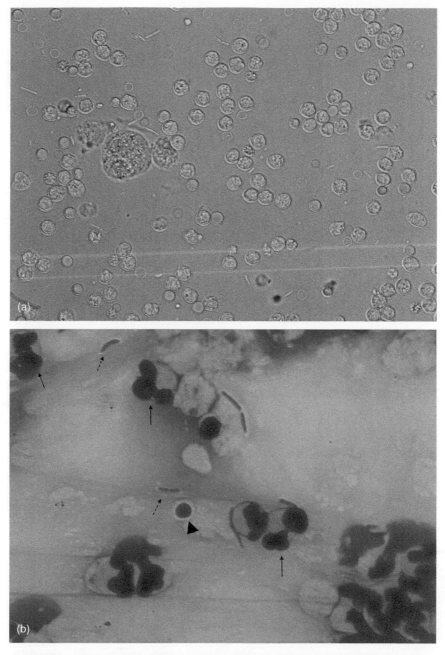

Figure 7.1 (a) Numerous WBCs, RBCs, few epithelial cells, and bacterial rods in urine sediment from a dog with a urinary tract infection, 40×; (b) air-dried and stained urine sediment. Neutrophils (arrows), bacterial rods (dashed arrows), and one yeast (arrowhead), Diff-Quick, 100×.

Urinary tract cytology

In some patients, urine cytology or aspiration of tissue (i.e. masses within the urethra, bladder, or kidneys) will provide more specific information regarding underlying disease(s). This is used most often to differentiate inflammation and infection from neoplasia or investigate mass lesions or organomegaly, if present.

Urine cytology

Urine cytology can be used to better characterize inflammatory cell types and infectious agents, differentiate types of epithelial cells, and evaluate criteria of malignancy within a population of cells. Urine cytology utilizes stained, air-dried urine sediment smears; the procedure described above is one method used to prepare a specimen for cytological evaluation. Preparation of the sediment itself takes gentle smearing as cells may be easily disrupted or distorted. Cytocentrifugation of urine or urine sediment offers superior preservation of cellular detail but requires special equipment found primarily in clinical pathology laboratories. Staining with Romanowsky-type stains (e.g. Diff-Quick or Wright Giemsa stain) allows for improved visualization of cells and infectious agents within a sample. The condenser must be raised to just under the stage to maximize cell detail in stained specimens. Urine is a harsh environment for cells, and rapid deterioration of nucleated cells can hinder attempts at cytological evaluation. Even when a urine specimen is processed quickly, the time the urine was present in the bladder may impact preservation. Cells exhibiting "urine scald" display enlarged, swollen nuclei with lacy chromatin, vacuolated cytoplasm, and irregular nuclear and cytoplasmic margins. Because of their irregularity, they may be mistaken for neoplastic cells (Figure 7.2a,b).

Clinical signs such as hematuria, pollakiuria, and stranguria, the presence of a mass at the trigone region of the bladder, a thickened urethra, or an enlarged prostate, or the presence of atypical cells in urine sediment may prompt cytological evaluation of urine to look for underlying neoplasia. Transitional (urothelial) cell carcinoma (TCC) is most common. TCC can develop from any portion of the urinary tract that is lined by transitional epithelial cells, including the urethra, bladder, ureters, and parts of the kidney. Non-neoplastic processes, that is, hyperplasia and dysplasia secondary to a UTI or benign polyps, may display increased epithelial cellularity but only mild pleomorphism as cells are mostly uniform in appearance (Figure 7.3a–c). Criteria of malignancy with TCC are often overt, and cytological diagnosis should be based on cytomorphologic abnormalities rather than clinical suspicion. Criteria of malignancy that are useful in diagnosing a TCC include significant anisocytosis (variation in cell size) and anisokaryosis (variation in nuclear size), preferably within the same cell cluster, increased nuclear to cytoplasm ratio (N:C) in large cells, bi- or multinucleation, anisokaryosis within the same cell, micronuclei, very large or angular nucleoli, and mitotic

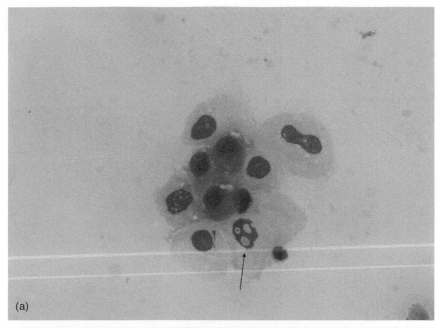

(a)

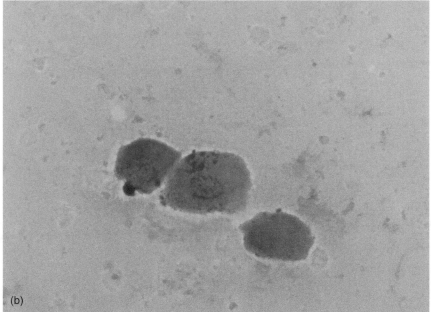

(b)

Figure 7.2 (a) Urine-scalded epithelial cells surrounding three more well-preserved cells. Note the swollen, lacy nuclei (arrow) and faint cytoplasm of the urine-scalded cells. Wright Giemsa, 50× (Courtesy of Dr. Reema Patel); (b) urine-scalded epithelial cells. The poor cellular preservation results from prolonged contact with urine, either in the bladder or due to a processing delay. Note the remaining outline of the nucleus, hazy cytoplasm, and irregular cytoplasmic margins. Wright Giemsa, 100×. (Courtesy of Dr. Reema Patel)

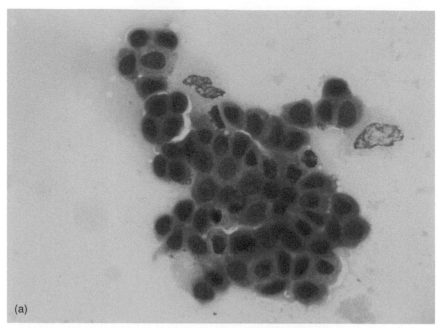

(a)

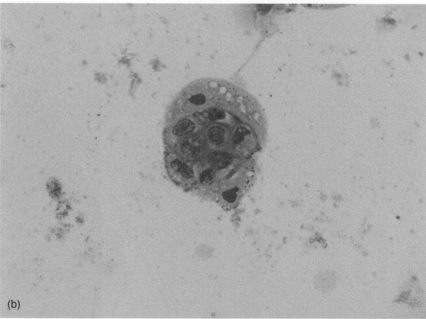

(b)

Figure 7.3 (a) Transitional epithelial cells. Hyperplasia of transitional epithelium may result from inflammation from infection or irritation (i.e. bladder stones) and polyps within the bladder. Although many cells are present, cells are fairly uniform in appearance. Wright Giemsa, 50× (Courtesy of Dr. Reema Patel). (b) Transitional epithelial cells. Although the N:C is increased, cell size and nuclear size are uniform, suggesting the dysplasia is a result of hyperplasia rather than neoplasia. Wright Giemsa, 50× (Courtesy of Dr. Reema Patel). (c) Transitional epithelial cells. This cluster of transitional epithelial cells exhibits the effects of prolonged exposure to urine given the swollen nuclei and cytoplasm. Wright Giemsa, 50×. (Courtesy of Dr. Reema Patel)

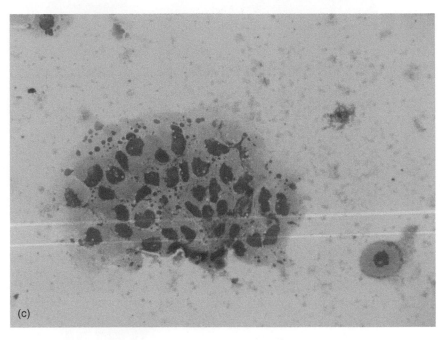

(c)

Figure 7.3 (*Continued*)

figures. Characteristic round to ovoid, magenta, stippled inclusions can sometimes be found in the cytoplasm of transitional epithelial cells. These inclusions are not pathognomonic for transitional (urothelial) cells as similar pink to magenta inclusions can also be identified in mesothelial cells. Their presence, however, in cells exhibiting significant criteria of malignancy in urine, certainly supports an interpretation of TCC (Figure 7.4a,b).

Lymphoma is also infrequently identified and can be present anywhere within the urinary tract. Lymphoma would be suspected if lymphoblasts were identified within a urine cytology specimen. Lymphoblasts are typically larger than a neutrophil with immature finely granular chromatin and visible nucleoli.

In some cases, urine cytology may not allow for definitive diagnosis, especially if the cells do not exfoliate easily (i.e. sarcomas) or if cell preservation in urine is poor. In these cases, traumatic catheterization of the mass is sometimes employed with slides prepared from either the resulting fluid and/ or impression smears of pieces of tissue. Percutaneous aspiration may also be performed; however, this procedure may result in seeding of the neoplasia, especially TCC, along the needle tract.

Renal cytology

A mass associated with a kidney or renomegaly, either uni- or bilateral, may necessitate aspiration. Aspiration is typically ultrasound-guided, although impression smears are sometimes prepared from biopsy samples or from

Chapter 7

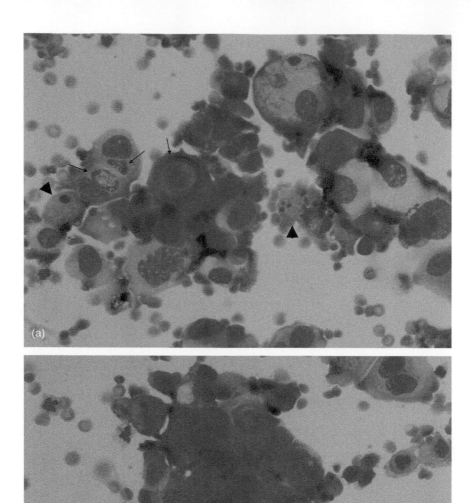

Figure 7.4 (a) and (b) Transitional (urothelial) cell carcinoma. Neoplastic transitional epithelial cells exhibit anisocytosis, anisokaryosis, bi- and multinucleation, immature ropy chromatin with visible nucleoli. Transitional epithelial cells may occasionally display characteristic magenta cytoplasmic inclusions (arrows). Several pyknotic cells also present (arrowheads), cytocentrifuged urine sample, Wright Giemsa, 40×.

deceased patients during necropsy. Normal structures that may be sampled and thus visualized include glomeruli, intact renal tubules, renal tubular epithelial cells, and potentially caudate transitional renal epithelial cells. It is important to recognize normal structures so not to incorrectly identify them as a pathological process (Figures 7.5–7.9).

Mass-like renal lesions can result from inflammation, cysts, or neoplasia. Depending on the extent and type of inflammation, aspiration may yield a variably cellular sample. Significant inflammation would warrant search for an underlying infectious etiology although cases of feline infectious peritonitis can reveal dramatic pyogranulatomous inflammation without an obvious etiology. In some cases such as renal abscesses or, less frequently, with pyelonephritis, evidence of inflammation may be apparent in the urine. Cystic lesions are usually of lower cellularity with a pink proteinaceous background; sometimes, macrophages, neutrophils, and erythrocytes are present in low numbers. Neoplastic processes can include both primary and metastatic lesions.

Renal lymphoma tends to produce highly cellular aspirates; either one or both kidneys as well as other organs may be affected. Cytological diagnosis is based on the presence of numerous lymphoblasts without a concomitant increase in plasma cells or other inflammatory cell types. Lymphoblasts can be recognized based on size (larger than a neutrophil), immature chromatin (finely granular to granular or stippled), and visible nucleoli. Lymphoblasts

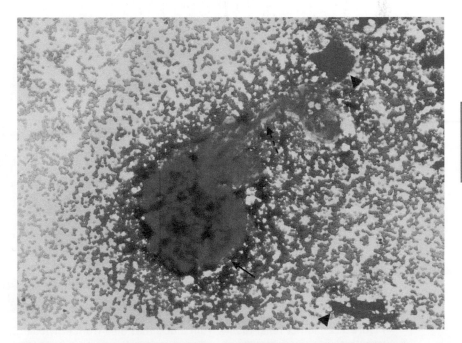

Figure 7.5 Intact glomerulus with a capillary tuft (arrow) and attached tubular epithelial cells (dashed arrow). Platelet clumps (arrowhead) and abundant background blood are also present. Wright Giemsa, 10×.

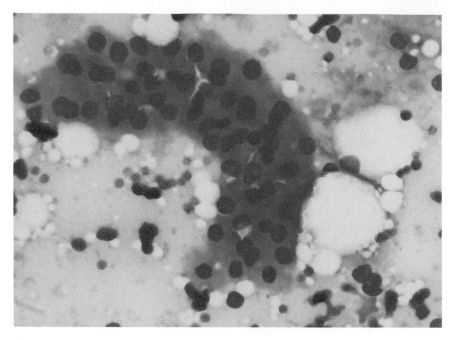

Figure 7.6 Higher magnificent view of an intact renal tubule from aspiration of a cat's kidney. Cells are cuboidal with uniform-appearing nuclei, clumped chromatin, and indistinct nucleoli. Cells can sometimes contain dark blue coarsely granular pigment. Wright Giemsa, 40×.

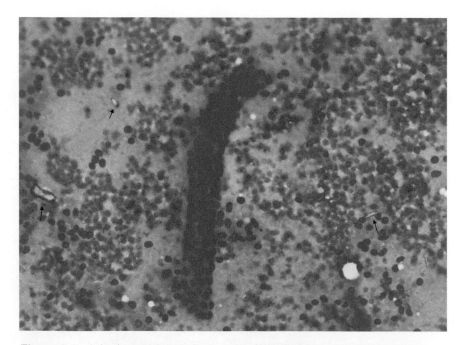

Figure 7.7 Intact renal tubule from a dog that died from ethylene glycol intoxication. Few crystals (arrows) are noted in the background along with abundant blood and bare nuclei from tubular epithelial cells. Wright Giemsa, 20×.

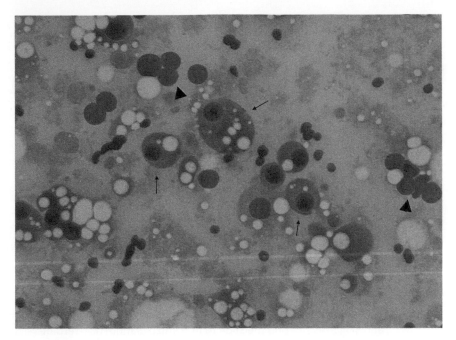

Figure 7.8 Renal tubular epithelial cells from a cat. Several variably sized epithelial cells (arrows), bare nuclei (arrowheads), RBCs, and free lipid. Note the epithelial cells frequently contain lipid vacuoles; this is a normal finding. Aqueous Romanowsky stain, 40×.

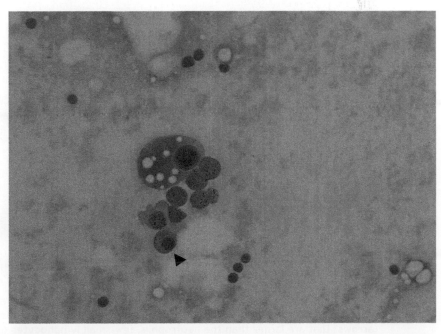

Figure 7.9 Renal tubular epithelial cell, plasma cell (arrowhead), bare nuclei, and RBCs. Aqueous Romanowsky stain, 40×.

must not be confused with bare nuclei or ruptured cells that quickly swell and display both an increased size and visible nucleoli (Figure 7.10).

Renal carcinoma can vary from well to poorly differentiated and typically presents as a unilateral mass or enlarged kidney. Cellularity is often high. Cells may retain their cuboidal to ovoid shape and be present individually, in clusters, or form tubular structures. Criteria of malignancy may be minimal to pronounced, depending on the degree of differentiation (Figures 7.11–7.13).

Summary of urinary tract cytology

If urinalysis results do not provide a conclusive explanation in patients where physical exam, clinicopathological data, or radiographic or ultrasonographic findings support underlying urinary tract disease, cytology of the urine or urinary tract can be an extremely useful diagnostic tool. Urine tract cytology does require an adequately preserved sample, proper sample preparation, and skill in evaluating the slide to maximize diagnostic usefulness. Submission of cytology specimens to an experienced cytopathologist is another option and may be helpful in characterizing abnormal cells or identifying potential organisms.

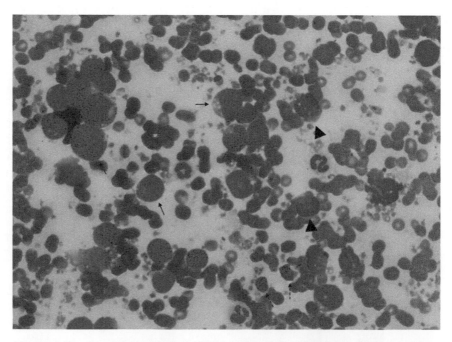

Figure 7.10 Renal lymphoma. Aspirates of an enlarged kidney from a patient with bilateral renomegaly. There is a predominance of large lymphoblasts (arrows) that are larger than the neutrophils, few small lymphocytes (dashed arrows), ruptured cells (arrowheads), many erythrocytes, abundant basophilic globular cytoplasmic debris, Wright Giemsa, 50×.

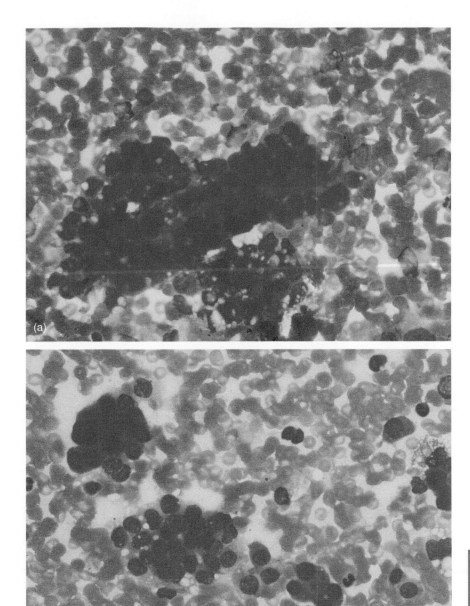

Figure 7.11 (a) and (b) Renal adenocarcinoma. Aspiration of a renal mass from a dog reveals large clusters of neoplastic epithelial cells that form tubular and acinar structures. Dark pink secretory product is present within tubular lumen and acini. Epithelial cells exhibit an increased nuclear to cytoplasm ratio, binucleation, anisokaryosis (variation in nuclear size), and visible nucleoli. Wright Giemsa, 40×.

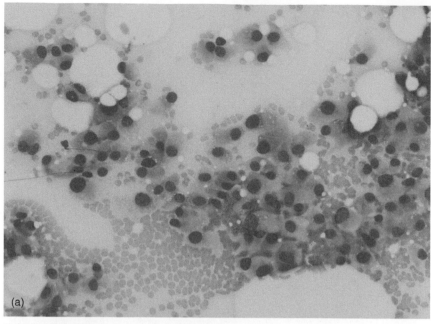

(a)

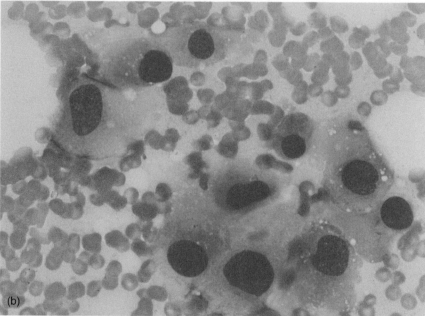

(b)

Figure 7.12   (a) Renal carcinoma. Highly cellular sample from aspiration of a renal mass in a dog. Cells are individualized to loosely cohesive. Cells bear some resemblance to normal renal tubular epithelial cells but exhibit an increased nuclear to cytoplasm ratio, anisokaryosis, binucleation, and some prominent large nucleoli. Wright Giemsa, 20×. (b) Renal carcinoma. Higher magnification view. Neoplastic epithelial cells exhibit anisocytosis (variable cell size), aniskaryosis with variably shaped nuclei, immature stippled chromatin, multiple nucleoli within the same nucleus, and giant nucleoli. Wright Giemsa, 50×.

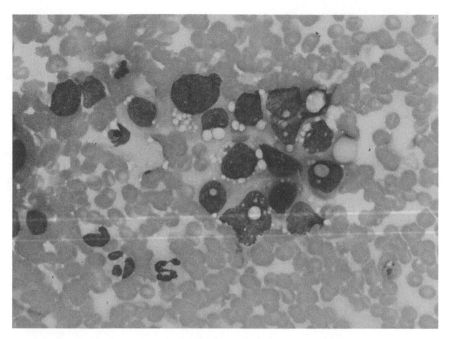

Figure 7.13 Renal carcinoma. Aspiration of a renal mass from a dog contains individual and clusters of neoplastic renal epithelial cells. Neoplastic cells exhibit a two- to threefold variation in nuclear size and some prominent, large nucleoli. This population contains lipid similar to the cells in Figure 7.6. Histopathology identified this mass as a tubular carcinoma. Wright Giemsa, 50×.

Fractional excretion

Fractional excretion (FE) of an analyte (FE_x), frequently an electrolyte, is determined by both glomerular filtration and tubular reabsorption. Electrolytes are freely filtered at the glomerulus and then can be reabsorbed or secreted by renal tubules. FE provides an estimate, expressed as a percentage, of the amount of analyte excreted in the urine, and so indirectly assesses the ability of the renal tubules to reabsorb an analyte. Plasma and urine concentrations of the analyte are compared to plasma and urine creatinine (Crt) values (Stockham and Scott 2008) (Eq. 7.1). As described for UPC, excretion of creatinine is relatively constant and allows for a single urine collection rather than a 24-hour urine collection, which is unrealistic in veterinary practice.

$$FE_x = \frac{X_{urine} \times Crt_{plasma}}{X_{plasma} \times Crt_{urine}}$$ (Eq. 7.1)

In general, if an analyte is freely filtered at the glomerulus and undergoes no tubular reabsorption or excretion, the same amount in the plasma and urine would be expected, that is, FE = 1. If some of the analyte were reabsorbed by

Chapter 7

Table 7.1 Considerations for interpretation of increased and decreased FE

Increased FE

    Increased urinary excretion of an analyte

        Plasma concentration of analyte are increased (kidneys excrete more)

        Decreased tubular reabsorption of analyte

        Increased tubular secretion of analyte

        Decreased creatinine excretion (i.e. decreased glomerular filtration rate [GFR])

Decreased FE

    Low plasma concentrations of analyte (kidneys then appropriately conserve analyte)

    Increased tubular reabsorption of analyte

    Decreased tubular secretion of analyte

Sources: Data from Lefebvre et al. (2008); Stockham and Scott (2008).

Table 7.2 Normal values for fractional excretion in dogs and cats

Analyte	Fractional excretion	
	Dogs	Cats
Sodium	<1%	<1%
Chloride	<1%	1.3%
Potassium	<20%	24%
Phosphorous	<39%	73%

Sources: Data from DiBartola (2000); Finco et al. (1992).

the renal tubules so that less remains in the urine than in the plasma, the FE is expected to be <1 (Stockham and Scott 2008) (Table 7.1).

FE is greatly influenced by preanalytical and analytical factors that may limit its usefulness (Braun et al. 2003; Lefebvre et al. 2008). Along with renal tubular function, age, breed, gender, diet, biological rhythms, and exercise can impact FE (Hoskins et al. 1991; Lane et al. 2000; Lefebvre et al. 2008; Lulich et al. 1991; Stevenson and Markwell 2001; Stockham and Scott 2008). FEs of sodium (FE_{Na}), chloride (FE_{Cl}), potassium (FE_K), phosphorous (FE_P), bicarbonate (FE_{HCO3}), and calcium (FE_{Ca}) are the analytes more often measured. "Normal" values ultimately depend on the patient's clinical status, and there can be a wide variability even within the same patient (Lefebvre et al. 2008). Also, changes in FE may not be a result of tubular dysfunction but rather a result of homeostasis and response to changing plasma concentrations (Finco et al. 1992). FE values should always be considered in light of patient clinical status, dietary and fluid intake, breed, age, and gender (Table 7.2).

Use of FE in veterinary medicine

The primary clinical use of FE is to identify renal tubular dysfunction, although normal FE values do not rule out disease. Both inherited (Fanconi's syndrome) and acquired diseases (nephrotoxic drugs, hypotension, infection) may result in renal tubular disease and increased loss of electrolytes into the urine. FE of electrolytes may help in determining the degree of renal disease in azotemic dogs (Buranakarl et al. 2007). FE_{Na} has been used in human medicine as well as veterinary medicine to differentiate prerenal causes of azotemia from acute tubular necrosis (Carvounis et al. 2002; Waldrop 2008). $FE_{Na} < 1\%$ is expected in cases of prerenal azotemia, that is, dehydration, while $FE_{Na} > 2\%$ is expected in severe acute tubular injury (Waldrop 2008). Unfortunately, this is highly variable, and FE results may not accurately categorize the underlying disease, especially when diuretics are used (Carvounis et al. 2002). Measurement of FE_{Na} has been recommended to monitor hypotension- or drug-induced (i.e. aminoglycoside antibiotics, amphotericin B, nonsteroidal anti-inflammatory drugs (NSAIDs), contrast media, and angiotensin-converting enzyme inhibitors) renal injury (Nolin and Himmelfarb 2010; Waldrop 2008). Although FE_{Na} can be impacted, changes may not reflect the degree of injury; better indicators of renal tubular injury should be relied upon to monitor drug-induced nephrotoxicity (Grauer et al. 1996; Rivers et al. 1996; Riviere et al. 1981). (See urinary biomarkers below.)

Urinary biomarkers

The proximal convoluted tubule, the first portion of the renal tubules receiving ultrafiltrate from the glomerulus, is responsible for reabsorption of numerous solutes including glucose, amino acids, electrolytes, urea, and water, and demonstrates high metabolic activity. It also functions to reabsorb and process some low and intermediate molecular proteins that are able to pass through the glomerular filter. Enzymes originating in renal tubular epithelial cells can be measured in urine and used as markers of renal tubular injury or dysfunction. N-acetyl-beta-D-glucosaminidase (NAG) and gamma-glutamyl transpeptidase (GGT) are located in the lysosomes and brush border, respectively, of the proximal convoluted tubule (Chemo 1998). Increases in enzymes GGT and NAG and certain low and intermediate molecular weight proteins in the urine can provide information regarding renal tubular injury and dysfunction.

Urine enzymology: Urine GGT and NAG

GGT is commonly measured in plasma or serum to test for hepatic or biliary disease, specifically cholestasis. GGT present in the plasma does not enter into the tubular filtrate due to an inability to cross the glomerular filtration barrier (Stockham and Scott 2008). Urine GGT, therefore, originates in renal tubular epithelial cells. NAG originates in the urinary tract, primarily the proximal renal tubular epithelial cells, and can be measured in urine. Urine concentrations of GGT and NAG are compared to urine creatinine concentrations to overcome the influence of urine specific gravity (USG) (Grauer et al. 1995). The comparison to urine creatinine provides a good estimate of 24-hour urinary excretion (Grauer et al. 1995). For either enzyme, a NAG or GGT index (U/g) or urine enzyme to creatinine ratio can be calculated based on the following equation (Eq. 7.2, Urine enzyme [GGT or NAG] index):

$$\text{NAG or GGT index (U/g)} = \frac{\text{Urine}_{enzyme} \text{ (U/L)}}{\text{Urine}_{crt} \text{ (g/L)}} \qquad \text{(Eq. 7.2)}$$

Increases in GGT and/or NAG index may precede increases in standard measures of renal disease especially in cases of acute tubular injury (Chemo 1998; Grauer et al. 1995; Greco et al. 1985; Rivers et al. 1996). An elevated NAG index, greater than normal or baseline values, has been reported in dogs with various diseases including chronic renal disease, leishmaniasis, and pyometra, as well as dogs treated with aminoglycoside antibiotics, glucocorticoids, and some NSAIDs (Grauer et al. 1995; Heiene et al. 2001; Sato et al. 2002a,b; Smets et al. 2010). Reference ranges or expected values for NAG and GGT indexes in normal dogs and cats have been published (Brunker et al. 2009; Sato et al. 2002a,b). Because of significant differences in urine NAG index between males and females, different normal ranges should be used for interpretation (Brunker et al. 2009). Also, pH can influence urinary GGT where a low urine pH can decrease GGT due to inactivation of the enzyme (Table 7.3).

In both dogs and cats with chronic renal disease, the NAG index was much higher than the value in normal animals (Sato et al. 2002a,b). In the patients with chronic renal disease, the NAG index ranged from 15.7 to 136.8 U/g in dogs and from 6.2 to 35.5 U/g in cat (Sato et al. 2002a,b). These increases preceded changes in BUN and creatinine. While urine GGT is available at some reference laboratories, NAG is mostly limited to research laboratories at this point as reference ranges and testing protocols are further refined. In the future, both tests may become more widely available.

Table 7.3   Proposed normal ranges for NAG and GGT

Index	Male	Female
NAG–Dogs	0.02-3.65 U/g	0.02-2.31 U/g
NAG–Cats	1.5 +/− 1.0 U/g	1.7 +/− 1.8 U/g
GGT–Dogs	1.93-28.57 U/g	

Sources: Data from Brunker et al. (2009); Sato et al. (2002a,b).

Urinary proteins as biomarkers for renal disease

The presence of increased amounts of certain proteins can be used to identify the presence and determine the magnitude of renal disease. As described in Chapter 6, "Proteinuria," glomerular filtration typically excludes larger proteins, including albumin, from entering into the tubular fluid. Proteins entering into the ultrafiltrate are reabsorbed, via specific receptors (i.e. megalin and cubilin), by proximal renal tubular epithelial cells. These proteins then undergo lysosomal degradation within the epithelial cells. An excess of filtered proteins, due to glomerular disease, a lack of reabsorption of proteins, due to overflow proteinuria or tubular disease, or both can result in proteinuria. Measurement of various low, intermediate, and high molecular weight proteins in urine can be used to assess renal function, specifically glomerular filtration and tubular reabsorption. This practice is more common in human nephrology although several veterinary studies have examined their usefulness (Forterre et al. 2004; Nabity et al. 2011; Smets et al. 2010; Vinge et al. 2010). In human nephrology, some biomarkers (both protein and nonprotein) considered useful for the diagnosis of acute kidney injury include NAG, retinol binding protein (RBP), kidney injury molecule-1 (KIM-1), urine and serum neutrophil gelatinase-associated lipocalin (NGAL), urinary interleukin-18 (IL-18), and liver-type fatty acid binding protein (Parikh et al. 2010). Some of these biomarkers have been evaluated in veterinary medicine in a research setting, but even in human nephrology, these are still under investigation (Parikh et al. 2010). Commercial tests may be developed as the methodologies and understanding move forward.

Albumin

Albumin, an intermediate weight molecular (IMW) protein, is the most commonly measured urine protein and remains a useful indicator of underlying glomerular and tubular disease. Microalbuminuria assays offer greater sensitivity and specificity over routine tests for urine protein; these assays are reviewed in Chapter 6. A urine albumin to creatinine ratio provides a quantitative measure of urine albumin; increases are seen with chronic kidney disease (Smets et al. 2010). Albuminuria can result from either tubular or glomerular injury or disease and so other biomarkers may offer a greater degree of specificity.

RBP

RBP is an LMW protein that is freely filtered at the glomerulus (Smets et al. 2010). Following entry into the tubular fluid, RBP is reabsorbed via specific receptors (i.e. megalin) within the proximal tubular epithelial cells (Christensen et al. 1998; Dillon et al. 1998; Forterre et al. 2004; Smets et al. 2010). Increases in RBP are seen in dogs with chronic renal disease and in hyperthyroid cats (Smets et al. 2010; Van Hoek et al. 2009). Increased urinary excretion of RBP precedes azotemia but not proteinuria in a canine model of inherited glomerular disease (Nabity et al. 2011).

Tamm–Horsfall protein

The absence of normally excreted proteins can also reflect renal tubular disease. Tamm–Horsfall protein (THP), also known as uromodulin, is secreted by distal tubular epithelial cells in dogs (Forterre et al. 2004). Trace and 1+ urine protein dipstick reactions sometimes observed in the highly concentrated urine specimens from dogs are attributed to THP, as well as other nonpathological proteins. Decreased renal excretion of THP was seen in dogs with renal disease and is hypothesized to be a specific indicator of distal renal tubular injury (Forterre et al. 2004). Routine testing for THP is not widely available.

Summary of biomarkers

The presence of increased amounts of urinary albumin, RBP, GGT, or NAG indicates renal injury and/or disease. The latter three are more specific of tubular disease although lack of reabsorption of low and intermediate molecular weight proteins can occur with glomerular disease due to competition for proximal renal tubular receptors. Currently, only urine albumin and urine GGT can be routinely evaluated, but continued research and test validation efforts will likely result in better and more widely available biomarkers to diagnose early or subclinical renal disease.

References

Bartges JW. 2004. Diagnosis of urinary tract infections. *Veterinary Clinics of North America. Small Animal Practice* **4**(4): 922-33.

Braun JP, Lefebvre HP, Watson AD. 2003. Creatinine in the dog: a review. *Veterinary Clinical Pathology* **32**: 162-79.

Brunker JD, Ponzio NM, Payton ME. 2009. Indices of urine N-acetyl-beta-D-glucosaminidase and gamma-glutamyl transpeptidase activities in clinically normal adult dogs. *American Journal of Veterinary Research* **70**(2): 297-301.

Buranakarl C, Ankanaporn K, Thammacharoen S, Trisiriroj M, Maleeratmongkol T, Thongchai P, Panasjaroen S. 2007. Relationships between degree of azotaemia and blood pressure, urinary protein : creatinine ratio and fractional excretion of electrolytes in dogs with renal azotaemia. 2007. *Veterinary Research Communications* **31**(3): 245-57.

Carvounis CP, Nisaw S, Guro-Razuman S. 2002. Significance of the fractional excretion of urea in the differential diagnosis of acute renal failure. *Kidney International* **62**(6): 2223-9.

Chemo FAS. 1998. Urinary enzyme evaluation of nephrotoxicity in the dog. *Toxicologic Pathology* **26**(1): 29-32.

Christensen EL, Birn H, Verroust P, Moestrup SK. 1998. Megalin-mediated endocytosis in renal proximal tubule. *Renal Failure* **20**(2): 191-9.

DiBartola SP. 2000. Clinical approach and laboratory evaluation of renal disease. In *Textbook of Veterinary Internal Medicine*, 5th ed. Ettinger SJ, Feldman EC, eds., pp. 1600-14. Philadelphia: WB Saunders.

Dillon SC, Taylor GM, Shah V. 1998. Diagnostic value of urinary retinol-binding protein in childhood nephrotic syndrome. *Pediatric Nephrology* **12**: 643-7.

Finco DR, Barsanti JA, Brown SA. 1992. Solute fractional excretion rates. In *Current Veterinary Therapy XI*. Kirk RW, Bonagura JD, eds., pp. 818-20.Philadelphia: WB Saunders.

Forterre S, Raila J, Schweigert FJ. 2004. Protein profiling of urine from dogs with renal disease using ProteinChip analysis. *Journal of Veterinary Diagnostic Investigation* **16**(4): 271-7.

Grauer GF, Greco DS, Behrend EN, Fettman MJ, Mani I, Getzy DM, Reinhart GA. 1996. Effects of dietary n-3 fatty acid supplementation versus thromboxane synthetase inhibition on gentamicin induced nephrotoxicosis in healthy male dogs. *American Journal of Veterinary Research* **57**(6): 918-56.

Grauer GF, Greco DS, Behrend EN, Mani I, Fettman MJ, Allen TA. 1995. Estimation of quantitative enzymuria in dogs with gentamicin-induced nephrotoxicosis using urine enzyme/creatinine ratios from spot urine samples. *Journal of Veterinary Internal Medicine* **9**(5): 324-7.

Greco DS, Turnwald GH, Adams R, Gossett KA, Kearney M, Casey H. 1985. Urinary gamma-glutamyl transpeptidase activity in dogs with gentamicin-induced nephrotoxicity. *American Journal of Veterinary Research* **46**(11): 2332-5.

Heiene R, Moe L, Molmen G. 2001. Calculation of urinary enzyme excretion, with renal structure and function in dogs with pyometra. *Research in Veterinary Science* **70**: 129-37.

Hoskins JD, Turnwald GH, Kearney MT, Gossett KA, Fakier N. 1991. Quantitative urinalysis in kittens from four to thirty weeks after birth. *American Journal of Veterinary Research* **52**(8): 1295-99.

Klausner JS, Osborne CA, Stevens JB. 1976. Clinical evaluation of commercial reagent strips for detection of significant bacteriuria in dogs and cats. *American Journal of Veterinary Research* **37**(6): 719-22.

Lane IF, Shaw DH, Burton SA, Donald AW. 2000. Quantitative urinalysis in healthy Beagle puppies from 9 to 27 weeks of age. *American Journal of Veterinary Research* **61**(5): 577-81.

Lefebvre HP, Dossin O, Trumel C, Braun JP. 2008. Fractional excretion tests: a critical review of methods and applications in domestic animals. *Veterinary Clinical Pathology* **37**(1): 4-20.

Lulich JP, Osborne CA, Polzin DJ, Johnston SD, Parker ML. 1991. Urine metabolite values in fed and nonfed clinically normal Beagles. *American Journal of Veterinary Research* **52**(10): 1573-8.

Nabity MB, Lees GE, Dangott LJ, Cianciolo R, Suchodolski JS, Steiner JM. 2011. Proteomic analysis of urine from male dogs during early stages of tubulointerstitial injury in a canine model of progressive glomerular disease. *Veterinary Clinical Pathology* **40**(2): 222-36. epub.

Nolin TD, Himmelfarb J. 2010. Mechanisms of drug-induced nephrotoxicity. *Handbook of Experimental Pharmacology* **1**(196): 111-30.

Parikh CR, Lu JC, Coca SG, Devarajan P. 2010. Tubular proteinuria in acute kidney injury: a critical evaluation of current status and future promise. *Annals of Clinical Biochemistry* **47**(4): 301-12.

Rivers BJ, Walter PA, O'Brien TD, King VL, Polzin DJ. 1996. Evaluation of urine gamma-glutamyl transpeptidase-to-creatinine ratio as a diagnostic tool in an

Chapter 7

experimental model of aminoglycoside-induced acute renal failure in the dog. *Journal of the American Animal Hospital Association* **32**(4): 323-36.

Riviere JE, Coppoc GL, Hinsman EJ, Carlton WW. 1981. Gentamicin pharmacokinetic changes in induced acute canine nephrotoxic glomerulonephritis. *Antimicrobial Agents and Chemotherapy* **20**(3): 387-92.

Sato R, Soeta S, Miyazaki M, Syuto B, Sato J, Miyake Y, Yasuda J, Okada K, Naito Y. 2002a. Clinical availability of urinary N-acetyl-beta-D-glucosaminidase index in dogs with urinary disease. *The Journal of Veterinary Medical Science* **64**(4): 361-5.

Sato R, Soeta S, Syuto B, Yamagishi N, Sato J, Naito Y. 2002b. Urinary excretion of N-acetyl-beta-D-glucosaminidase and its isoenzymes in cats with urinary disease. *The Journal of Veterinary Medical Science* **64**(4): 367-71.

Smets PM, Meyer E, Maddens BE, Duchateau L, Daminet S. 2010. Urinary markers in healthy young and aged dogs and dogs with chronic kidney disease. *Journal of Veterinary Internal Medicine* **24**(1): 65-72.

Stevenson AE, Markwell PJ. 2001. Comparison of urine composition of healthy Labrador Retrievers and Miniature Schnauzers. *American Journal of Veterinary Research* **62**(11): 1782-6.

Stockham SL, Scott MA. 2008. Urinary system. In *Fundamentals of Veterinary Clinical Pathology*, 2nd ed. Stockham SL, Scott MA, eds., pp. 426-33. Ames, IA: Blackwell Publishing.

Swenson CL, Boisvert AM, Kruger JM, Gibbons-Burgener SN. 2004. Evaluation of modified Wright-staining of urine sediment as a method for accurate detection of bacteriuria in dogs. *Journal of the American Veterinary Association* **224**(8): 1282-9.

Tivapasi MT, Hodges J, Byrne BA, Christopher MM. 2009. Diagnostic utility and cost-effectiveness of reflex bacterial culture for the detection of urinary tract infection in dogs with low urine specific gravity. *Veterinary Clinical Pathology* **38**(3): 337-42.

Vaden SL, Levine J, Breitschwerdt EB. 1997. A retrospective case-control of acute renal failure in 99 dogs. *Journal of Veterinary Internal Medicine* **11**(2): 58-64.

Van Hoek I, Lefebvre HP, Peremans K, Meyer E, Croubels S, Vandermeulen E, Kooistra H, Saunders JH, Binst D, Daminet S. 2009. Short- and long-term follow-up of glomerular and tubular renal markers of kidney function in hyperthyroid cats after treatment with radioiodine. *Domestic Animal Endocrinology* **36**(1): 45-56.

Vinge L, Lees GE, Nielsen R, Kashtan CE, Bahr A, Christensen EI. 2010. The effect of progressive glomerular disease on megalin-mediated endocytosis in kidney. *Nephrology, Dialysis, Transplantation* **25**(8): 2458-67. epub.

Waldrop JE. 2008. Urinary electolytes, solutes, and osmolality. *Veterinary Clinics North America. Small Animal Practice* **38**(3): 503-12.

Chapter 7

Chapter 8
Laboratory Quality Assurance

Quality laboratory performance is a culmination of planned events executed through daily activities of management and staff. This chapter offers suggestions to accentuate performance in any clinical laboratory setting. Compliance with local, state, and federal codes is always mandatory and supersedes any advice set forth in this chapter.

Physical requirements of the laboratory

Laboratory design and arrangement

A well-designed laboratory utilizes space efficiently, following equipment specifications and recognizing the needs of laboratory personnel (Lifshitz et al. 2007). Those with general knowledge of space requirements should be involved in the design plan along with consultants, architects, and engineers as necessary. With full input to the process, laboratory workers can benefit from creating a safe work environment that is functional and aesthetically pleasing (Mortland and Mortland 2010).

Work zones created by grouping equipment and instruments sharing the same function together optimize laboratory performance. For example, a microscope, centrifuge, dipstick reader, laboratory information workstation, and sink in close proximity streamline the workflow for the urinalysis section. Likewise, storage for reagents and disposables nearby minimizes time needed to replenish these items. Ergonomically compliant benches, shelving, cabinets, chairs, and keyboard drawers reduce the risk of repetitive stress injuries to staff (www.labortorydesign.com).

Laboratory space allotted to house all equipment and personnel must satisfy occupancy and fire codes. Broad isles and walkways facilitate staff retreat in case of emergency; furniture or equipment cannot impede egress. Wide doorways simplify equipment delivery and removal; floors must be constructed to bear the weight load of the items and staff contained therein.

Practical Veterinary Urinalysis, First Edition. Carolyn Sink, Nicole Weinstein.
© 2012 John Wiley & Sons, Inc. Published 2012 by John Wiley & Sons, Inc.

Chapter 8

Spaces between cabinets, benches, and equipment permit access for cleaning and allow enough room for maintenance and service of equipment. A variety of cabinet configurations can accommodate bulk storage or daily supplies needed at technical workstations (www.laboratorydesign.com).

Climate control

Instrument specifications provide guidelines and restrictions on room temperature and humidity. If installed, fume hoods cannot be the only means of room exhaust. If windows are incorporated in the laboratory design for ventilation purposes, they should be lockable and contain insect screens. Regulatory guidelines specify the number of air exchanges needed per hour (www.stanford.edu/dept/EHS.prod).

Electrical requirements

One of the obvious electrical needs for the laboratory is an adequate number of electrical receptacles which are properly configured for equipment. Additionally, the reviewing electrical demand of each item ensures proper generating capacity to satisfy demand and avoid power failure. Dedicated electrical circuits may be needed for sensitive equipment or for those necessitating high electrical demand. Line filters may be used to eliminate random fluctuation of an electrical signal. An uninterruptible power supply (UPS) provides temporary power when the main power source fails; UPS are battery powered and typically provide power for 5–15 minute duration. When used in conjunction with an emergency power generator, laboratory functionality can be maintained during catastrophic power failure.

Electronic communication

Planning should include adequate number of data lines strategically located throughout the laboratory. An adequate number of data lines strategically located throughout the laboratory promotes efficiency. Anticipating demands of future technologies assures success in transition to new applications when needed.

Water and plumbing

Laboratory instrumentation often dictates the type of water needed in the clinical laboratory. For smaller pieces of equipment, reservoirs containing the appropriate water type may be purchased to accommodate analysis but for larger pieces of equipment or for laboratory equipment with high demand, "feedwater" may be purified on site. Clinical and Laboratory Standards Institute (CLSI) defines six grades of water purity each requiring specific components and filters (Table 8.1). Additional steps may be needed to purify

Table 8.1 Clinical and Laboratory Standards Institute (CLSI) water types

CLSI water type	Intended use
Autoclave and wash water	Feedwater for autoclave and/or automatic laboratory dishwashers with heated dry cycles
Commercially bottled, purified water	Laboratory must validate water for acceptable performance for testing throughout period of use
Water supplied by method manufacturer for use as a diluent or reagent	Specified on product label
Instrument feedwater	Internal rinse, dilution, and water bath functions of automated analyzers
Clinical laboratory reagent water	Most routine laboratory analysis
Special reagent water	Trace organic or mineral analysis, DNA and RNA testing, cell/tissue/organ cultures

Source: Data from Miller et al. (2006).

feedwater with high mineral content or unique contaminates (Miller et al. 2006; Sunheimer et al. 2007).

Laboratory wastewater should be discharged in compliance with regulatory specifications. In the event wastewater is accumulated for disposal, provisions should be made to house receptacles in laboratory areas to avoid spills (www.stanford.edu/dept/EHS.prod).

Drench hoses, sink faucets, or bath showers are not suitable eyewash facilities; safety showers and eyewash stations should be highly visible, well lit, and possess a clear path of access (www.ehss.vt.edu).

Laboratory equipment

Equipment acquisition

Vendors are eager to place their analyzers in your laboratory. Staking this claim typically ensures continued purchase of reagents, parts, and consumables in addition to payment for instrument service. A wide variety of financial options are available to obtain laboratory equipment including, but not limited to, outright purchase, lease, or rental. The financial need of the organization should be considered when committing to one of these methods of instrument acquisition. The same option may not be preferable for every purchase (Travers 1997) (Table 8.2).

Outright purchase of equipment is advantageous if full ownership of the instrument is the goal. A comprehensive cost analysis may prove helpful to

Chapter 8

Table 8.2 Methods of equipment acquisition

Acquisition type	Advantages	Disadvantages
Cost per reportable	Pay only for reportable tests	Reportables may include repeats, quality control, or calibration
Rental	Flexible usage time Hedge obsolescence	May be costly in the long term
Financial lease	Full ownership at end of term Acquire equipment otherwise unobtainable	Payment of interest or financing cost Noncancelable agreement
True lease	Flexible financing Option to include reagents and related supplies	Nonownership Interest payment or financing costs
Purchase	Full ownership	Large capital outlay Technical obsolescence over time Additional costs of reagents and supplies

Sources: Data from Jaros et al. (2007); Travers (1997).

justify purchase. Once an asset, the equipment may be viewed as a depreciation expense and will most likely not be included in monthly budgetary documents. Disadvantages of instrument purchase are large capital outlay in addition to risk that the technology purchased becomes obsolete prior to the organization recovering the instrument purchase price through sale of laboratory tests (Jaros et al. 2007; Travers 1997).

An advantage of an operating (true) lease is that obsolescence is hedged since the agreement is typically cancelable. Additionally, this method of instrument acquisition offers flexibility in financing. With an operating lease, the full responsibility for the instrument is with the owner; repairs, reagents, and related supplies are usually included in the lease price. The lessee may or may not have a purchase option at completion of the lease agreement and should be considered when entering a true lease. Major disadvantages of the operating lease are nonownership of the equipment and payment of interest or financing costs (Travers 1997).

Like the operating lease, the financial lease usually includes interest or financing costs, but unlike the true lease, the organization usually will own the equipment at the end of the lease agreement. This noncancelable agreement offers organizations that are short on capital outlay an opportunity to acquire laboratory equipment that may otherwise be unobtainable (Travers 1997).

Equipment rental offers flexibility in usage time; an organization may enter into monthly or annual rentals. An ideal method to hedge obsolescence, equipment rental may prove to be costly in the long term. Some vendors offer a reagent rental program that provides the instrumentation at "no cost" but increase reagent prices that ultimately provide instrument payment (Jaros et al. 2007).

Some vendors allow instrument acquisition through cost per reportable option; only the fees for reportable or billable tests are paid to the vendor. Buyer beware! Repeats, calibration, and quality control samples may be included, thus increasing the overall cost of this option.

Equipment for urinalysis

Veterinary refractometers

Reichert Rhino VET360 refractometer (Depew, NY) is a handheld unit containing three scales that can determine protein concentration in serum, plasma, or peritoneal fluid, urine specific gravity for cats, urine specific gravity for dogs and large animals. One drop of fluid on the prism allows the user to take a reading by holding the refractometer toward a light source.

Misco Vetmed Refractomter (Cleveland, OH) is a portable digital unit also containing three scales that can determine protein concentration in serum, plasma, or peritoneal fluid, urine specific gravity for cats, urine specific gravity for dogs and large animals. One drop of fluid provides results through a digital readout.

Centrifuges

Centrifuge size often dictates selection, and many bench top units are available for purchase. Smaller units may be noisier than larger ones, so decibel output should be examined if the unit will reside in a confined area in the lab. A swing bucket rotor head provides leveled sediment and is preferred over a fixed head rotor that produces an angled sediment meniscus.

Microscopes

A high-quality light microscope with 10× and 40× objectives is necessary for reading urine sediment. A tilting binocular head provides adjustment to suit individual preference and comfort. If sediment imaging is desired, a digital camera can be attached through a photo tube.

Electronic reagent strip readers

Visual interpretation of dry reagent strips used for urinalysis testing is prone to error as laboratory personnel are required to discern different shades of a color reaction. To improve consistency, electronic reagent strip readers may be employed. These readers consist of a sliding tray or feed mechanism that automatically move the urine saturated strip into a reading head at timed intervals using reflectance technology; recent models aspirate a specific amount of urine, deposit it on a test strip, and read at appropriate intervals by reflectance. Typically, only one configuration of dry reagent strips may be used at a time. Depending on the manufacturer, throughput ranges from 7 to 70 seconds per strip. Results are available for print or download to an information system.

Reagents and supplies for the urinalysis laboratory

Reagents and supplies

It is imperative to optimize laboratory inventory levels to accommodate testing need. This can be a daunting task, as test demand may be unpredictable. Reagent and supply inventory is the responsibility of all who utilize the lab; however, the task of ordering reagents or supplies may be assigned to one individual to avoid duplication of orders. If the test volume is constant and there is no staff member dedicated to inventory management, it may be beneficial to enroll in "standing orders" to provide automatic delivery of laboratory related items. This may reduce shipping costs and alleviate some burden of monitoring stock levels.

Some vendors may offer volume discounts for laboratory reagents, but the monetary benefit may be negated if testing is never actualized. As some inventory may expire before use, staff should be encouraged to use short-date reagents and supplies first. Short-date items should be strategically located throughout the lab so that they are easily placed in the user's hand. Reagents and supplies must also be stored in the correct environment so that external factors do not render the product useless prior to testing.

Commonly used supplies in the urinalysis laboratory

Sorbent wipes
$3'' \times 1'' \times 1mm$ Microscope slides
$22 \times 22mm$ Cover glass or 10-well constant volume chamber
Disposable pipettes

Commonly used reagents in the urinalysis laboratory

5% Sulfosalicylic acid in dropper bottle
10% Sodium hydroxide in dropper bottle
10% Hydrochloric acid in dropper bottle

Laboratory waste

Biohazardous waste

Biohazardous materials include veterinary biologicals and animal pathogens. Biohazards generated from the laboratory should be disposed of according to regulatory statures. For the most part, any biological agent that is

Chapter 8

suspected of or known to cause disease in humans or animals should be disposed of through a waste stream that prohibits the spread of the disease or infectious agent (www.ehss.vt.edu).

Chemical waste

Many reagents used in the laboratory are considered hazardous chemicals; thus management must employ methods devised to minimize personnel exposure to hazardous products. Compliance with the Occupational Safety and Health Administration (OSHA) regulations is expected in an effort to prevent harmful exposure to hazardous materials in the workplace. Manufacturers are required to provide recommendations for safe storage, use, and disposal of hazardous materials which they sell. This is accomplished by distribution of Material Safety Data Sheets (MSDSs). MSDSs should be readily available for laboratory staff review and daily use (www.ehss.vt.edu).

Sharps

Any fine point capable of cutting or piercing the skin or an autoclave bag is considered a sharp. This includes needles, scalpel blades, glass slides, blood collection tubes, and pipettes. Sharps should be disposed of in a puncture proof container according to regulatory guidelines (ehss.vt.edu).

Quality control in the urinalysis laboratory

Quality control for refractometers

Refractometer performance should be verified daily with at least two levels of control materials. Assayed quality control materials are available commercially. Readings outside acceptable levels may mandate refractometer adjustment through calibration. Distilled water provides an inexpensive zero calibrator; 5% sodium chloride (1.022 ± 0.001) and 9% sucrose should (1.034 ± 0.001) provide mid- and high-level calibrators (Strasinger and DiLorenzo 2008). Daily quality control readings should be recorded in instrument-specific quality control records along with calibration adjustments.

Quality control for dry reagent strips

A wide variety of assayed quality control material for dipsticks is available; a few are listed in Table 8.3. Each laboratory should choose a product best suited to its need. Often, these materials are also assayed for specific gravity and can be used for quality assessment of refractometer(s) and confirmatory test methods. Dipstick performance should be tested on a daily basis. Results outside expected values should be investigated and may mandate disposal of defective strips.

Chapter 8

Table 8.3 Popular assayed quality control materials for urine dipsticks

Name	Type	Analytes
Bio-Rad Liquichek™	Liquid, human urine based	Bilirubin, blood, creatinine, glucose, ketones, leukocyte esterase, microalbumin, microscopics, nitrite, osmolality, pH, protein, specific gravity, urobilinogen
Quantimetrix Dipper™	Liquid, human urine based	Bilirubin, blood, creatinine, glucose, ketones, leukocyte esterase, microalbumin, nitrite, pH, protein, specific gravity, urobilinogen
Siemens CHECK-STIX™	Firm plastic strips with six separate dry reagent areas affixed Requires reconstitution in deionized water	Bilirubin, blood, glucose, ketone (acetoacetic acid), leukocyte esterase, nitrite, pH, protein, specific gravity, urobilinogen

Quality control for technical staff

Assayed quality control materials are available for assessing quality of microscopy. Redundancy of reading the same material day after day may not challenge staff expertise, so it may be advantageous for management to instead issue "homemade" challenge specimens on a daily, weekly, or monthly basis. Specimens containing both normal and abnormal findings are recommended.

Quality standards for centrifugation

Any centrifuge used in the urinalysis section should be configured to accept specimen tubes used for dipstick analysis. A swinging bucket centrifuge head renders the specimen sediment level within the specimen tube; capped specimens should be centrifuged at 400 × g for 5 minutes. Centrifugation time in revolutions per minute (RPM) should be calculated using this formula:

$$RPM = (\text{square root } (400/28.38R)) \times 1000$$

where R = radius of centrifuge rotor in inches (Sink and Feldman 2004).

All members of the laboratory team should utilize the same centrifuge while employing identical centrifugation time and speed for urine sediment preparation.

Table 8.4 Format for individual procedures contained in a procedure manual

Section	Explanation
Title	Name of the procedure Cite commonly used abbreviations
Purpose	Reason for laboratory analysis Include clinical relevance of the procedure
Specimen	List acceptable specimen(s), including preservatives or anticoagulants
Equipment/reagents/ supplies	Inclusive list Provide instructions for reagent preparation
Quality control	Detail quality control material(s) and appropriate use
Procedure	Describe procedure step-by-step
Results	Provide raw data analysis or calculations used to derive result Specify units for reporting result
Reference(s)	Provide primary literature reference(s)

Procedure manuals

A procedure manual is a compilation of documents that contain step-by-step instructions for a given discipline. In the clinical laboratory, procedure manuals are typically grouped according to subspecialty, that is, chemistry, hematology, urinalysis. Individual procedures contained within serve as reference documents and when followed by technical personnel, assure consistency of a repetitive task and reproducible test results.

The procedure manual is provided by management but written by a laboratory expert for technical personnel. All established methods utilized within the laboratory should be appropriately documented. A catalog of laboratory "how-tos," the procedure manual may be available in paper or electronically but should reside at the laboratory testing bench to be used for frequent reference.

The format of the procedure manual should be consistent; a suggested format for individual procedures is found in Table 8.4. In addition to technical procedures, protocols for daily, weekly, and monthly standard operating procedures (SOPs) should be included to cite management's expectations for execution of tasks (Flatland et al. 2010). These SOPs may reference a variety of procedures including instrument maintenance, stock replenishing, and inventory control.

It is important to understand the difference between procedure and protocol. A procedure contains sequential instruction to perform a given task. A protocol is a system of rules that govern a procedure or procedures and

Chapter 8

overview function of a given laboratory task. A well-written procedure manual should contain both by referencing laboratory procedures within the corresponding protocol.

Procedure manuals are only effective when those performing a specific task follow instruction. For this reason, it is imperative that staff is involved in formulating the documents contained and provide input to detail within. Updating procedure manuals is necessary, including annual review, revision, or retirement of procedures as they are outdated or replaced. Likewise, new procedures and protocols should be added to the procedure manual as needed.

References

Flatland B, Freeman KP, Friedrichs KR, Vap LM, Getzy KM, Evans EW, Harr KE. 2010. ASVCP quality assurance guidelines: control of general analytical factors in veterinary laboratories. *Veterinary Clinical Pathology* **39**(3): 264-77.

Jaros ML, Lifshitz MS, De Cresce RP. 2007. Financial management. In *Henry's Clinical Diagnosis and Management by Laboratory Methods*, 21st ed. McPherson RA, Pincus MR, eds., pp. 122-33. Philadelphia: Saunders.

Lifshitz MS, DeCresce RP, Lutinger I. 2007. Optimizing laboratory workflow and performance. In *Henry's Clinical Diagnosis and Management by Laboratory Methods*, 21st ed. McPherson R. A., Pincus MR, eds., pp. 12-9. Philadelphia: Saunders.

Miller WG, Gibbs E, Jay D, Pratt K, Rossi B, Vojt C, Whitehead P. 2006. *Preparation and Testing of Reagent Water in the Clinical Laboratory: Approved Guideline*, 4th ed. Wayne, PA: Clinical and Laboratory Standards Institute.

Mortland K, Mortland D. 2010. Lean architectural basics for labs. *Advance for Medical Laboratory Professionals* **22**(13): 6-8.

Sink CA, Feldman BF. 2004. *Laboratory Urinalysis and Hematology for the Small Animal Practitioner*. Jackson, WY: Teton NewMedia.

Strasinger SK, DiLorenzo MS. 2008. Quality assessment and management in the urinalysis laboratory. In *Urinalysis and Body Fluids*, 5th ed. Strasinger SK, DiLorenzo MS, eds., pp. 127-42. Philadelphia: FA Davis.

Sunheimer RL, Threatte G, Lifshitz MS, Pinus MR. 2007. Analysis: principles of instrumentation. In *Henry's Clinical Diagnosis and Management by Laboratory Methods*, 21st ed. McPherson R. A., Pincus MR, eds., pp. 56-63. Philadelphia: Saunders.

Travers E. 1997. Technology acquisition. In *Clinical Laboratory Management*. Mitchell CW, ed., pp. 333-73. Philadelphia: Lippincott Williams & Wilkins.

Webliography

www.laboratorydesign.com/public/labtopics.html Information on fume hoods, air conditioning, and chemical storage for laboratories.

www.stanford.edu/dept/EHS/prod/ Information on general laboratory safety topics.

www.ehss.vt.edu/ Information on general laboratory safety.

Index

Note: Entries with "f" indicate figures; those with "t" indicate tables.

Practical Veterinary Urinalysis, First Edition. Carolyn Sink, Nicole Weinstein.
© 2012 John Wiley & Sons, Inc. Published 2012 by John Wiley & Sons, Inc.